# Islamic Approaches to Patient Care

Muslim Beliefs and Healthcare Practices for Caregivers

# Islamic Approaches to Patient Care

## Muslim Beliefs and Healthcare Practices for Caregivers

Ra'ufa Sherry Tuell

amana publications

First Edition
(1432AH/2011AC)


amana publications
10710 Tucker Street
Beltsville, Maryland 20705-2223 USA
Tel: (301) 595-5777 / Fax: (301) 595-5888
E-mail: amana@igprinting.com
www.amana-publications.com

Library of Congress Cataloging-in-Publication Data

Tuell, Ra'ufa Sherry.
Islamic approaches to patient care : Muslim beliefs and healthcare practices for caregivers / Ra'ufa Sherry Tuell.
p. cm.
Includes bibliographical references.
ISBN 978-1-59008-070-2
1. Medicine--Religious aspects--Islam. 2. Medical care. 3. Islam--Customs and practices. 4. Caregivers--Handbooks, manuals, etc. I. Title.
BP166.72.T84 2011
297.2'66--dc23
2011026890

Printed in Turkey By Mega Print

# IN DEDICATION

To Sidi Shaykh Muhammad Sa'id al-Jamal ar-Rifa'i ash-Shadhuli, the guide of the peace, the mercy, and the love to the way of Allah through the Sufi path of the Shadhdhuliyyah Tariqah, the head of the Higher Sufi Council in Jerusalem and the Holy Land, and teacher and central figure at Masjid al-Aqsa in Jerusalem

"Allah created all people from dust for they are equal and must follow the heavenly teaching and the message of all the Prophets. The Prophets are all brothers, and their Lord is one, and their Creator and their message is one. All come from one father and mother."

- Sidi Shaykh Muhammad Sa'id al-Jamal ar-Rifa'i ash-Shadhuli,
the Farm of Peace, Warfordsburg, Pennsylvania, September 2008

*Islamic Approaches to Patient Care — Muslim Beliefs and Healthcare Practices for Caregivers was written under the supervision of Ingrid Mattson, Ph.D., professor and director of the Duncan Black Macdonald Center for the Study of Islam and Christian-Muslim Relations at Hartford Seminary in Hartford, Conn. The book also was reviewed by Mohamed Magid, president of the Islamic Society of North America, and the executive director of the All Dulles Area Muslim Society (ADAMS) in Washington, D.C.*

# ABSTRACT

The need to understand the religion of Islam from the perspective of Muslim patients is real and compelling, as Islam is now the fastest growing religion in America. *Islamic Approaches to Patient Care: Muslim Beliefs and Healthcare Practices for Caregivers* is a step in that direction. It provides an overview of Islam's birth and early history, of the diverse Muslim population in the U.S., and of the basic beliefs and practices of worship. It also covers Islamic law and medical ethics and explains the healthcare sensitivities of Muslims. The book focuses on the healthcare perspectives of Muslim – based on the precepts of the Qur'an, as practiced by the Prophet of Islam, Muhammad (*Sunna*), and on the opinions of Islamic scholars, jurists, and organizations. No mention is made of any particular Muslim culture. The healthcare perspectives covered are abortion, autopsy, female and male circumcision, death and dying, euthanasia, suicide and assisted suicide, fertility regulation, infertility treatment, organ transplantation, and stem cell research. Lastly, ten appendices provide practical guidelines for facilitating the burial preparation of deceased Muslims, welcoming a newborn baby, a collection of commonly used prayers and expressions, online resources, and a glossary of terms.

وَإِذَا سَأَلَكَ عِبَادِي عَنِّي فَإِنِّي قَرِيبٌ أُجِيبُ دَعْوَةَ الدَّاعِ إِذَا دَعَانِ فَلْيَسْتَجِيبُواْ لِي وَلْيُؤْمِنُواْ بِي لَعَلَّهُمْ يَرْشُدُونَ

"And if My servants ask thee about Me – behold,
I am near; I respond to the call of him who calls,
whenever he calls unto Me: let them, then,
respond unto Me, and believe in Me,
so that they might follow the right way."

— Qur'an 2:186

# ACKNOWLEDGMENTS

To Allah, The Creator and The Sustainer

To the many people who supported the making of *Islamic Approaches to Patient Care: Muslim Beliefs and Helathcare Practices for Caregivers* including (in alphabetical order), Mahmoud Ayoub, Ph.D., Phyllis Lautz Biddle, Steven Blackburn, Ph.D., Sarah Stasha Christian, Claudia Hamda Coke, Bobbie Muniba Harlow Combe, Emile Latif Combe, Ph.D., Kim Fitzsimons, Alan Godlas, Ph.D., and Betty Godlas, Emily G. Holcombe, M.Div., J.D., Nura Carrie Khan, R.N., L.Ac., Hesham El-Meligy, John Wadude Laird, M.D., Imam Mohamed Magid, Reza Mansoor, M.D., Fatima Martin, Ph.D., Ingrid Mattson, Ph.D., Ivor Roberts, Aysha Saeed, M.D., John Swift, Rel.D., Judith Warn, CPS, and M.T. Winter, Ph.D.

To Aminah Assilmi (d. 2010), may God's mercy be upon her, for expertly steering this book to correctness in the way of Islam.

# TABLE OF CONTENTS

# INTRODUCTION

Providing compassionate care that supports people of every faith, or no faith, is at the heart of what healthcare professionals do. However, the expansion of Islam – now one of the fastest-growing religions in America[1] – has made this endeavor for non-Muslim healthcare professionals more challenging. The goal of this resource is to make it less so, and to provide those caring for Muslims with the tools and resources to support these patients.

*Islamic Approaches to Patient Care: Muslim Beliefs and Healthcare Practices for Caregivers* familiarizes readers with the basics of Islam. Because there are variations beyond these core elements, as is the case with all major religious traditions, much care was taken to speak in the broadest terms possible. Thus, the healthcare perspectives presented here may differ from those of an individual or culture. Moreover, a Muslim's response to serious illness, loss, and bereavement also depends on his or her emotional and spiritual state.

Additionally, this book addresses specific issues. Why do Muslims respond as they do to devastating traumas? What is the double-edged truth about death? Why are many Muslims accepting of chronic illnesses? Why do many Muslim women refuse abortions? How do medical breakthroughs cause ethical dilemmas for Muslim patients? This book provides realistic, fictitious scenarios to facilitate understanding of these and other healthcare issues. However, these scenarios are not meant to be all-inclusive, and understandably so, because the array of complicated healthcare issues is beyond the scope of this endeavor.

The sources for this book include readings on Islam and participation in seminars and classes about Islam at Hartford Seminary, Hartford, Conn. Other sources include interviews with non-Muslim and Muslim chaplains and physicians, with Muslim patients, and with clerics (*imams*, which means "those who stand in front") and scholars of Islam. The writer also draws on her experiences as a Muslim hospital chaplain.

The primary sources with regard to standards of conduct and character used in the book are the Qur'an, the sacred scripture of Islam, and the actions and words of Prophet Muhammad (*Sunna*) from a collection of reports (*ahadith*). Interpretations of these sources by learned scholars also are cited throughout the book. The Qur'anic English translation is that of Muhammad Asad's *The Message of the Qur'an*.[2]

Special notes about this book:

1. The name of God in Arabic is Allah. This term comes from the definite article of "the" (*al*) and deity (*'ilah*) and is commonly used by Muslims and Arabic-speaking Christians and Jews. The terms God and Allah are used interchangeably in this book.
2. The Arabic language does not capitalize letters.
3. The terms Sunni, Sunnites, or Sunnism refer to the largest branch of Islam; whereas, the terms Shia, Shiite, or Shiism refer to the second largest branch.

4. Muslims invoke the Qur'an's injunction of remembering the name of Prophet Muhammad by saying *sall Allahu 'aly-hi wa-sallam* (May Allah honor him and grant him peace) immediately after mention of his name whether in script, thought, or aloud. Qur'an 33:56: "Verily, God and His angels bless the Prophet: [hence,] O you who have attained to faith, bless him and give yourselves up [to his guidance] in utter self-surrender!" Muslims also invoke similar blessings for other prophets, angels, and for the name of God. These various blessings are implied within the text of this book.

NOTES

[1] David Roozen, "A Quick Question: How quickly are Muslim mosques growing in the U.S.?" at the website of Hartford Seminary, http://hirr.hartsem.edu/research/quick_question20.html. Accessed 8 January 2010.

[2.] Muhammad Asad, trans., *The Message of the Qur'an* (Gibraltar: Dar al-Andalus Limited, 1980).

CHAPTER I

# OVERVIEW OF ISLAM FOR THE HEALTHCARE SETTING

## Birth and Early History of Islam

A person who professes Islam is a Muslim. The word Islam derives from the three Arabic root letters of *sīn-lām-mīm*. These root letters carry such multiple meanings as safety, security, freedom, immunity, escape, peace, submission, obedience, and gentleness.[1]

Muslims progressively experience these deeper meanings of their religion by surrendering to God and living according to the tenets of their faith. These tenets are set forth in the Qur'an, Islam's holiest text, and are exemplified in the actions and words (Sunna) of Prophet Muhammad. Qur'an 3:85 says, "For, if one goes in search of a religion other than self-surrender unto God, it will never be accepted from him, and in the life to come he shall be among the lost."

Although most Muslims believe Islam has been the religion of the prophets back to Adam, Islam as a religion began around 610 C.E.[2] It was then, Muslims believe, that the illiterate 40-year-old merchant Muhammad ibn Abdullah (b. 570 C.E./d. 632 C.E.), while on spiritual retreat in a desert mountain cave (Mount Hira) near his home in Mecca, first received a revelation, conveyed through the Angel Gabriel from God.

This was the first of many such messages, which, in their entirety, constitute the Qur'an. It also was the beginning of the role of Muhammad as a prophet. According to Qur'an 33:40, "[And know, O believers, that] Muhammad is not the father of any one of your men, but is God's Apostle and the Seal of all Prophets. And God has indeed full knowledge of everything."

In 615 C.E., the Prophet Muhammad began preaching publicly the message of the Qur'an in Mecca, the center of commerce, culture, and polytheism in the Arabian Peninsula. He called upon people to worship Allah alone ("Allah" is the Arabic name for God; it means "the one and only God")[3] and to care for orphans, the needy, and the poor. He warned that Hell awaits the sinners and Heaven the righteous and that God will hold everyone accountable for their words and deeds on the Day of Judgment. He preached that God sent the Qur'an to all humankind as a reminder that they, and all of creation, are dependent upon God, that God is All-Merciful, All-Compassionate, and All-Powerful, and that humanity's purpose is to worship and serve God, and to care for each other and all of creation. A primary goal of the Qur'an is to motivate people to establish a just and ethical social order on earth.[4]

Understandably, the polytheistic and hedonistic Meccans opposed Prophet Muhammad. His message challenged their beliefs, polytheistic-based economy, unjust social order, and licentiousness.[5] The Meccans struck back, killing and torturing many Muslims. Prophet Muhammad and his community of Muslims escaped in 622 C.E. to Yathrib (known today as Medina, Saudi Arabia). Yathrib tribal leaders earlier had invited the Prophet to bring peace and order to their large, fractious farming community, located 250 miles north of Mecca. The Muslim community's flight to Yathrib, known as the *hijra* (emigration), marks year one of the Islamic lunar calendar.

In 630 C.E., eight years after the *hijra*, Prophet Muhammad and thousands of Muslims marched on Mecca. Quickly, the Meccans capitulated. The Muslims took no revenge, and most Meccans converted to Islam. Prophet Muhammad then ejected the idols from *Al-Ka'ba* (a house of worship reported to have been built by prophets Abraham and Ishmael), and rededicated it to God. He returned to Medina and two years later, in 632 C.E., fell ill and died. By then, most of the population of the Arabian Peninsula had converted to Islam, and the tribes had united.

### Muslims in Brief

In 2001, the atrocity of 9/11 created unprecedented media coverage. Despite the glut of attention, a survey conducted by Gallup and the Coexist Foundation[6] reports that most Americans know little about the 1,400-year-old religion and, for that matter, Muslims – who they are, where they live, and what they believe.

A common stereotype is that all Muslims are Arabs and live in the Middle East, but this is incorrect. In reality, only one in five Muslims is Arab. Most Muslims live in Bangladesh, India, Indonesia, Nigeria, and Pakistan. Many live in Europe and America. According to the Pew Forum on Religion & Public Life's "Mapping of the Global Muslim Population," "While Muslims are found on all five inhabited continents, more than 60% of the global Muslim population is in Asia and about 20% is in the Middle East and North Africa. However, the Middle East-North Africa region has the highest percentage of Muslim-majority countries. Indeed, more than half of the 20 countries and territories in that region have populations that are approximately 95% Muslim or greater. More than 300 million Muslims, or one-fifth of the world's Muslim population, live in countries where Islam is not the majority religion. These minority Muslim populations are often quite large. India, for example, has the third-largest population of Muslims worldwide. China has more Muslims than Syria, while Russia is home to more Muslims than Jordan and Libya combined."[7]

Today's Muslim population in the world stands at about 1.57 billion, "representing 23% of an estimated 2009 world population of 6.9 billion."[8] In the U.S., the exact number of Muslims is unknown because the U.S. Census does not track religious affiliation. This absence of reliable data is why estimates of America's Muslim population vary — ranging from more than 1.3 million to 7 million.[9]

The American Muslim community is diverse. According to a 2009 Gallup survey of Muslim-Americans, more than 35 percent are African-American and 28 percent are Caucasian. About 18 percent are Asian, and the remaining identify as belonging to other races.[10] Large concentrations of Muslims reside in California, Illinois, Indiana, Michigan, and New York.[11]

Islam is one of the fastest-growing religious groups in America.[12] Many demographers say that the number of Muslims in the U.S. has outgrown the total number of Christian Scientists, Episcopalians, Jehovah's Witnesses, Mennonites, Mormons, Presbyterians, Quakers, Seventh-day Adventists, and Unitarians. Some say that Islam has surpassed, or is surpassing, the nation's second most commonly practiced religion, Judaism.[13] The largest Christian religion in the U.S. is the Roman Catholic Church. "It claims nearly 37 percent of all religiously affiliated people – 23 percent of the total population."[14]

The number of mosques also is increasing rapidly. In 1930, there were only 19 mosques in the U.S. By 1960, this number had risen to 230, and by 1980, it had reached 600.[15] As of 2000, a national survey counted 1,209 mosques.[16] Today, the number of mosques is second only in growth to Christian megachurches. "Mosques trailed megachurches, 83 percent of which grew by ten percent or more in membership from 1995 to 2000 as compared to 60 percent of masjids [Muslim congregations], which grew by 10 percent or more in that same time period," says David Roozen, director of the Hartford Institute for Religion Research and co-coordinator of the Faith Communities Today study.[17] Additionally, as of the year 2000 (the latest information available), there were 400 Islamic schools, 400 Islamic associations, and more than 200 Islamic publications, journals, and weekly newspapers in the United States.[18] Though united by the Islamic faith, Muslims are divided by theological branches. About 85 percent identify as Sunni and 15 percent as Shiite. Primarily, these two branches differ on who were the rightful successors of Prophet

Muhammad (b. 570 C.E. /d. 632 C.E.). In the seventh century, most Muslims said only the most qualified person (ruler or *caliph*) should lead the young Islamic nation politically. They became known as the Sunni. Other Muslims said that Prophet Muhammad had named his successor, 'Ali ibn Abu Talib, his cousin and son-in-law. They became known as the Shiite. To this day, Shiites believe that only the direct descendants of Prophet Muhammad should be the leaders (Imams) of the Muslim people. Note: Shiites believe these religious leaders are divinely appointed; thus, their title, "*Imam*," is capitalized in English translations.[19]

Lastly, Sufism is the mystical or esoteric dimension of Islam. Sufis believe in the unity of God. They focus on the presence of God in all of creation. They believe that the duality and seeming contradictions of the temporal plane of existence occlude the spiritual awareness of people, causing them to believe they are separate from God and God's love. Sufis are devoted to a life of spiritual study, deep spiritual meditation, and self-discipline. Through various inward-focused practices, such as chanting and praying, they strive for experiential knowledge (gnosis) of God. Sufi mystics are mostly Sunni and some are Shiite, and, as Muslims, they ascribe to and practice Islamic doctrine and follow religious law.[20] Sufis belong to assorted orders, such as the Shadhdhuliyyah Sufi Order, which originated in the seventh century in Morocco and today has more than five million followers worldwide. Other well-known Sufi orders include the Naqshbandi, centered in Istanbul, Turkey, Manchester, England, and the U.S.; the Mevlevi, also known as the Whirling Dervishes, founded in Konya, Turkey, by the followers of 13th-century Persian mystic-poet

Rumi; and Chishti, prominent in India and Pakistan. In America, some people call themselves Sufis, but they do not profess to be Muslims, and as such, do not believe in the doctrines of or participate in the worship practices of Islam.[21]

Muslims also ascribe to religious schools of jurisprudence. Within each school, Islamic jurists study the Qur'an and the Sunna (actions and words of Prophet Muhammad) to render legal opinions (*fatwas*) that are adhered to by their followers. The major Sunni schools of jurisprudence are Hanafi, Hanbali, Maliki, and Shafi'i. The main Shia school of jurisprudence is the Twelver-Imam (*Ithna 'Ashariyya*). Twelver-Imam adherents believe there are only twelve divinely ordained Imams, starting with 'Ali ibn Abu Talib, the son-in-law and cousin of Prophet Muhammad. The smaller Shia groups, Ismailis and Zaydis, believe there are seven and five Imams, respectively.

Sunni and Shia Muslims may be observant or non-observant Muslims. They may be fundamentalist, mainstream, reformist, cultural, or secular. Differences among these groups are philosophical, ideological, and cultural and are based on social context.

Broadly speaking, fundamentalist Muslims lean toward a more literal emulation of the faith practices of Prophet Muhammad and his closest companions of the seventh century C.E. Fundamentalist Muslim men, for example, may wear long robes and grow long beards, while Muslim women may cover their entire body, including the face. These Muslims stress returning to the fundamentals of Islam. They are mostly apolitical.

Mainstream U.S. Muslims are not homogenous. Rather, they are distinguished by a high degree of integration into the general American population. There is little-to-no cultural disparity between them and other Americans. They are mostly middle-class in outlook, education, and income. Typically, mainstream Muslims are observant. This means, for instance, that they may abstain from eating pork and drinking alcohol and attend weekly congregational prayers on Friday. Many mainstream Muslim American women may wear a headscarf (*hijab*).

Reformist or "progressive" Muslims say their views are in line with Islamic teachings; however, most Muslims disagree. This small minority group wants to change traditional teachings and practices of the Muslim community, arguing, for example, that Muslim women should be imams of mixed-gender congregations and Muslim homosexuals should be allowed to marry.

Cultural Muslims practice Islam the way they practice Islam in their countries of origin. Often, mosques are the major centers of interaction for cultural Muslims.

Secular Muslims are not inclined to participate in religious practices at the mosque. Their religious interactions largely occur through Islamic rituals specific to such occasions as birth, death, and marriage.

Islam is a religion of peace, reconciliation, and tolerance. There is, however, a very small group of religious extremists, identifying as Muslims, engaged in violent activities. These extremists are not associated with any particular organization, sect, or religious school of thought in Islam. Their violent activities are not based in Islamic tenets. Furthermore, their violent activities are condemned by prominent Muslim religious figures worldwide.[22]

## Islam's Diversity

American Muslims are distinctive and diverse. They have no one culture or lifestyle. The cultural heritages of Muslims, up to seven million in the U.S., are from nearly every country on earth. Their cuisines, traditions, languages, dress, and commemorations of religious holidays vary considerably. Although this book cannot cover the thousands of cultural ways that believers worldwide practice Islam, they need to be understood by those caring for the Muslim patients.

While scholars may teach that cultural practices are not Islam, many Muslims do not make a distinction between their culture and religion.

For example, some Muslim men grow beards, while others do not. Some wear an ankle- or knee-length loose-fitting garment, but many wear Western attire.

The mode of dress of Muslim women also varies. They may wear a headscarf (*hijab*), a full-body dress (also called *hijab*) with a face covering (*niqab*), or conservative westernized dress. Generally, female Muslims (*Muslimas*) dress simply and modestly.

Many Muslim women and men, especially those from immigrant communities, may be uncomfortable looking directly into the eyes of a person of the opposite gender. This is not a sign of disrespect or disdain for the other person, but rather a sign of respect for the Qur'an, which commands both men and women to lower their gaze. In Qur'an 24:30, God says: "Tell the believing men to lower their gaze and to be mindful of their chastity: this will be most conducive to their purity – [and,] verily, God is aware of all that they do." Moreover, Qur'an 24:31 says: "And tell the believing women to lower their gaze and to be mindful of their chastity, and not to display their charms [in public] …" Consequently, Muslim men and women avoid making physical contact with the opposite gender except with their respective spouses or close relatives. They generally avoid shaking hands. Occasionally, they do not share elevator or car rides or attend mixed-gender gatherings. Some never attend such gatherings, but others do. In the West, most Muslims act according to their own conscience in such awkward situations as shaking hands in business meetings.

American Muslims also are politically diverse and may vote, for example, Republican, Democrat, or Green Party. As is the case with other Americans, there is considerable variation in educational levels and occupations. Some Muslims are physicians, for instance, while others are merchants and homemakers.

Despite these broad ranges of differences, Muslims are united deeply by the core beliefs and worship practices of Islam. With regard to the core beliefs, both the Sunni and Shia Muslims believe in one God (monotheism), the prophets and messengers of God, in the divinely revealed scripture, the Day of Judgment, and angels. The Sunnis, however, believe in a sixth article of faith, destiny or fate (*qadar*). Sunni and Shia Muslims also are united in their adherence to the five worship practices of Islam: the declaration of faith (*shahadah*), ritual prayer (*salah*), almsgiving (*zakah*), fasting (*sawm*), and pilgrimage (*hajj*). A discussion about Islam's core beliefs and worship practices follows in chapters two and three of this book.

NOTES

[1] Edward William Lane, *An Arabic-English Lexicon* (London: Williams and Norgate, 1863-93), 1412.

[2] C.E. stands for "common era," a year-numbering system used worldwide in non-Christian cultures and in most contemporary religious studies and academia. The numbering system is identical to the one historically used by Christians for B.C. / A.D. B.C. stands for "before Christ." A.D. stands for Anno Domini, indicating the years after the birth of Jesus. The parallel to B.C. in the non-Chrisitian system is B.C.E., "before the common era."

[3] Umar Faruq Abd-Allah, "One God, Many Names," A Nawawi Foundation Paper, http://www.nawawi.org/downloads/article2.pdf. Accessed 6 April 2010.

[4] Fazlur Rahman, *Major Themes of the Qur'an* (Minneapolis, Minnesota: Bibliotheca Islamica, 1989), 1-6 and 37-64.

[5] Houston Smith, *Islam: A Concise Introduction* (New York: HarperCollins, 2001), 14.

[6] "The Muslim West Facts Project," a not-for-profit partnership between Gallup and the Coexist Foundation survey of religious attitudes of and about Muslims worldwide, conducted in 2008, http://www.muslimwestfacts.com/mwf/125318/Religious-Perceptions-America.aspx. Accessed 6 April 2010.

[7] Pew Forum on Religion & Public Life, "Mapping the Global Muslim Population," October 7, 2009, http://webcache.googleusercontent.com/search?q=cache:w_JnWS85ZuUJ:pewforum.org/WorkArea/linkit.aspx%3FLinkIdentifier%3Did%26ItemID%3D6305+mapping+the+global+muslim+population+pew&cd=1&hl=en&ct=clnk&gl=us&source=www.google.com. Accessed 22 May 2010.

[8] Ibid.

[9] Margaret A. Miklancie, "Caring for Patients of Diverse Religious Traditions: Islam a Way of Life for Muslims," in *Home Healthcare Nurse* 25, No. 6 (June 2007): 414. Miklancie attributes this statistic to "Pipe, 2001; American Religious Identity Survey [ARIS], 2001; 'Balancing Religious Sensitivity,' 2005."

[10] Mohamed Younis, "Muslim Americans Exemplify Diversity, Potential," http://www.muslimwestfacts.com/mwf/116266/Muslim-Americans-Exemplify Diversity-Potential.aspx. Accessed 6 April 2010.

[11] Ibid.

[12] David Roozen, "A Quick Question: How quickly are Muslim mosques growing in the U.S.?" at the website of Hartford Seminary, http://hirr.hartsem.edu/research/quick_question20.html. Accessed 8 January 2010.

[13] Jonah Blank, "The Muslim Mainstream," in *U.S. News,* July 20, 1998, http://www.jannah.org/articles/usnews.html. Accessed 9 January 2010.

[14] John Wright, ed., *The New York Times Almanac 2002* (New York: Penguin, 2001), 403.

[15] Muhammad Anwar, "Muslims in the West: demographic and socio-economic position," in *Caring for Muslims Patients*, 2nd ed., eds. Aziz Sheikh and Abdul Rashid Gatrad (Oxon, United Kingdom: Radcliffe Publishing, 2009) (hereinafter referred to as *Caring for Muslim Patients*), 9. Anwar attributed the above-cited information to Khalidi O (2000) Mosque, in Roof, W.C., ed., *Contemporary Religion* (New York: Macmillan, n.d., n.p.).

[16] Ibid. Same attribution as above.

[17] Roozen, ibid.

[18] Abdel Raheem Odeh Yosef, "Health Beliefs, Practice, and Priorities for Health Care of Arab Muslims in the United States," *Journal of Transcultural Nursing* 19, No. 3 (July 2008): 284. Note that Yosef attributed this information to the "Council on Islamic Education [CIE], 2000."

[19] Michael Cooperson, *Classical Arabic Biography: the heirs of the prophets in the age of al-Ma'mun* (Cambridge: Cambridge University Press, 2000), xx.

[20] The terms Sunni, Sunnite, or Sunnism refer to the largest branch of Islam; whereas, the terms Shia, Shiite, or Shiism refer to the second largest branch.

[21] Jamal Malik and John R. Hinnells, *Sufism in the West* (New York: Routledge, 2006), 12.

[22] Alan Godlas, "Islam and Islamic Studies," http://webcache.googleusercontent.com/search?q=cache:Z4vip4ZsGg8J:www.uga.edu/islam/+alan+godlas&cd=1&hl=en&ct=clnk&gl=us. Accessed 6 April 2010.

## CHAPTER 2

# THE SIX DOCTRINES OF BELIEF

Essential to Islam and required of all Muslims, is the belief in the doctrines of faith. For Sunni Muslims, these doctrines are the belief in the unity of God (*tawhid*), in angels, in the prophets and messengers of God, in the revealed books of God, in the Day of Judgment, and in divine destiny. It is the same for Shia Muslims; however, they do not ascribe to the belief in divine destiny (*qadar*).

### Belief in the Unity of God

Muslims proclaim this belief minimally five times daily in the declaration of faith or *shahadah* during the ritual prayer (*salah*). The first half of the shahadah states: "*ash-hadu an la ilaha illa Llah*" ... or "I witness that there is no god but God." This statement captures the core belief of Islam: monotheism. Qur'an 1:1-4 says, "Say: 'He is the One God: God the Eternal, the Uncaused Cause of All Being. He begets not, and neither is He begotten; and there is nothing that could be compared with Him.'" Furthermore, in Qur'an 4:36, God says, "...worship God [alone], and do not ascribe divinity, in any way, to aught beside Him." The second part of the declaration of faith states: "... *wa ash-hadu anna Muhammadan rasulu Llah*" or "and I witness that Muhammad is the Messenger of God." This part of the *shahadah* "registers the Muslim's faith in the authenticity of [Prophet] Muhammad and in the validity of the book (Qur'an) that he transmitted."[1] Saying the *shahadah* in front of two witnesses is all that is required to become Muslim.

### Belief in the Angels

Angels, Muslims believe, are created from light, are pure creatures, and cannot disobey God. They do have assigned tasks, however. Some angels only praise God. Others deliver messages from God to the prophets and messengers. The most notable messenger angel in Islam is Gabriel.[2] Muslims believe that Angel Gabriel transmitted the entire Qur'an – word for word for twenty-three years – from God to Prophet Muhammad.

Additionally, angels protect people. Qur'an 13:11 says, "(a person) has hosts of helpers – both such as can be perceived by him and such as are hidden from him – that could preserve him from whatever God may have willed."

Moreover, every person has two angels that record his/her deeds, starting at puberty[3] and ending at death. The angel on a person's right notes a Muslim's good actions, and the angel on the left notes the bad actions. On the Day of Judgment, one of the angels places the weightier of the books in the right or left hand of the person. The book in the left hand indicates the person is going to Hell; whereas, the book in the right hand means the person is going to Heaven. In Qur'an 50:16-18, God says:

> Now, verily, it is We who have created man, and We know what his innermost self whispers within him: for We are closer to him than his neck-vein. [And so,] whenever the two demands [of his

> nature] come face to face, contending from the right and from the left, not even a word can he utter but there is a watcher with him, ever-present.

Believing there is no place that a person can hide his or her deeds from God fosters a growing awareness of God (*taqwa*). God says in Qur'an 49:13, "O men! Behold, We have created you all out of a male and a female, and have made you into nations and tribes, so that you might come to know one another. Verily, the noblest of you in the sight of God is the one who is most deeply conscious of Him. Behold, God is all-knowing, all-aware."

### Belief in the Prophets and Messengers of God

There are many more prophets than messengers, as the latter bring a "scripture" to their people, in addition to their oral teaching, guidance and leadership.[4] Qur'an 2:136 says:

> We believe in God, and in that which has been bestowed from on high upon us, and that which has been bestowed upon Abraham and Ismail and Isaac and Jacob and their descendants, and that which has been vouchsafed to Moses and Jesus; and that which has been vouchsafed to all the [other] prophets by their Sustainer: we make no distinction between any of them. And it is unto Him that we surrender ourselves.

Muslims believe that Prophet Muhammad was the messenger sent by God to proclaim God's unity (*tawhid*), and as such was the final messenger of God. Islam embraces the other prophets without distinction. The Qur'an mentions twenty-five, including Abraham, Moses, and Jesus. Throughout the ages, their purpose was to convey God's revelations to people and "to guide humanity to the Straight Path of God."[5] It is important to note that Muslims honor Jesus as a prophet but reject his divinity.

### Belief in the Revealed Books of God

Muslims believe in the God-revealed books of the Torah (Moses), Psalms (David), and Gospel (Jesus). Qur'an 3:3-4 says:

> Step by step has He bestowed upon thee from on high this divine writ, setting forth the truth which confirms whatever there still remains [of earlier revelations]: for it is He who has bestowed from on high the Torah and the Gospel aforetime, as a guidance unto mankind, and it is He who has bestowed [upon man] the standard by which to discern the true from the false. Behold, as for those who are bent on denying God's messages – grievous suffering awaits them: for God is almighty, an avenger of evil.

For Muslims, God's book is the Qur'an.

> And unto thee [O Prophet] have We vouchsafed this divine writ, setting forth the truth, confirming the truth of whatever there still remains of earlier revelations and determining what is true therein. Judge, then, between the followers of earlier revelation in accordance. (Qur'an 5:48)

It is believed by Muslims to be the "purest extant scripture on earth, because it has been preserved from tampering."[6] God protects the Qur'an:

"Behold, it is We Ourselves who have bestowed from on high, step by step, this reminder: and, behold, it is We who shall truly guard it [from all corruption]." (Qur'an 15:9)

## Belief in the Day of Judgment

The Day of Judgment (*Yawm al-Qiyama*) occurs when the world ends, at the time of "The Darkening." According to Qur'an 81:1-14:

> When the sun is shrouded in darkness, and when the stars lose their light, and when the mountains are made to vanish, and when she-camels big with young, about to give birth, are left untended, and when all beasts are gathered together, and when the seas boil over, and when all human beings are coupled [with their deeds], and when the girl-child that was buried alive is made to ask for what crime she had been slain, and when the scrolls [of men's deeds] are unfolded, and when heaven is laid bare, and when the blazing fire [of hell] is kindled bright, and when paradise is brought into view: [on that Day] every human being will come to know what he has prepared [for himself].

Muslims believe that all of humankind will stand trial at the Day of Judgment, and according to the weight of their righteous and unrighteous thoughts, actions, and deeds, will be dispersed either to Heaven (*janna*) or Hell (*jahannam*). Each person will know his/her placement in the Hereafter by according to which angel places the record of deeds in which hand. If the record is placed in the right hand, the person is bound for janna or in the left hand the person is going to *jahannam*. Some Muslims believe that Prophet Muhammad will intercede with God on their behalf on the Day of Judgment. Others do not.

## Belief in the Divine Decree and Destiny

For centuries and to this day, Islamic scholars have debated the issue of divine decree and destiny (*al-qada wal-qadar*). Differences of opinion, therefore, are aplenty.

Essentially, however, *al-qada* (decree) loosely translates as measurement and pertains to the unfolding of creation, which according to the will and knowledge of God, is decreed in pre-eternity. The physical laws of the universe, such as the law of planetary motion and human genetics, are examples of *qada*. Qur'an 54:49 says: "Behold, everything have We created in due measure and proportion…" Therefore, Muslims believe that God alone created all of creation and that God alone endowed all aspects of creation with specific attributes and abilities.

On the other hand, the term *qadar* (destiny) pertains to the fruition of God's will. Most Muslims believe that God recorded everything in *The Preserved Book*, which is kept with Him in Heaven. A report (*hadith*) of Prophet Muhammad says, "God recorded the fates of all creatures 50,000 years before creating the heavens and the earth, and His throne was upon the water."[7] Furthermore, Qur'an 57:22 says, "No calamity can ever befall the earth, and neither your own selves, unless it be [laid down] in Our decree before We bring it into being: verily, all this is easy for God."

There are various interpretations of *qadar*. Some say that a person's ultimate fate is predetermined, regardless of his/her thoughts, actions, and deeds. Others disagree. They argue that it is impossible to know. This is not to say that *qadar* influences human choices. God gave humans free will, and because God is omniscient, He has full knowledge of what people are going to do even before they do. People are free to choose their reactions and responses to whatever comes their way. Nevertheless, the Qur'an encourages humans to strive constantly for proximity to God, regardless of circumstance, and says that both ease and hardship are opportunities for spiritual and emotional growth. Some Muslims believe that nothing happens but by the will or permission of God.

It must be noted that most Shia Muslims do not believe in divine destiny; however, Sunni Muslims do.

NOTES

[1] Houston Smith, *Islam: A Concise Introduction* (New York: HarperCollins, 2001), 49.

[2] Qur'an *Baqara* 2:97-98: "Say [O Prophet]: 'Whosoever is an enemy of Gabriel' - who, verily, by God's leave, has brought down upon thy heart this [divine writ] which confirms the truth of whatever there still remains [of earlier revelations], and is a guidance and a glad tiding for the believers -: 'whosoever is an enemy of God and His angels and His message-bearers, including Gabriel and Michael, [should know that,] verily, God is the enemy of all who deny the truth.'"

[3] Muslims believe that the age of accountability commences at puberty.

[4] Qur'an 3:3-4: "Step by step has He bestowed upon thee from on high this divine writ, setting forth the truth which confirms whatever there still remains [of earlier revelations]: for it is He who has bestowed from on high the Torah and the Gospel - aforetime, as a guidance unto mankind, and it is He who has bestowed [upon man] the standard by which to discern the true from the false. Behold, as for those who are bent on denying God's messages - grievous suffering awaits them: for God is almighty, an avenger of evil."

[5] Hammudah Abdulati, *Islam in Focus*, rev. ed., eds. Shaykh Salih al Husayin and Dr. Mustapha Abu Sway (Beltsville, MD: amana publications, 1998), 11.

[6] Frederick Mathewson Denny, *An Introduction to Islam*, 2nd ed. (New York: Macmillan, 1994), 108.

[7] Denny, 112. The author cited as the following source of this *hadith*: Al-Baghawi, *Mishkat al-Masabih*, trans. James Robson (Lahore, Pakistan: Sh. Muhammad Ashraf, 1965-1966), vol. 1, 23.

## CHAPTER 3

# THE FIVE PILLARS OF PRACTICING ISLAM

Muslims practice the five rituals or "pillars" of their faith. These pillars, which are mandatory for Muslims, are the declaration of faith (*shahadah*), the ritual prayer (*salah*), the almsgiving (*zakah*), the fast (*sawm*), and the pilgrimage (*hajj*).

### The Declaration of Faith (*Shahadah*)

In Arabic, the *shahadah* states: "*ash-hadu an la ilaha illa Llah wa ash-hadu anna Muhammadan rasulu Lah*" or "I witness that there is no god but God, and I witness that Muhammad is the Messenger of God." This affirmation is the most spoken testimony of faith in the Islamic world. Minimally, Muslims say the *shahadah* at prayer (*salah*) five times daily, and they gently whisper the *shahadah* into the ears of the newborn and the dying. They also say the *shahadah* many times throughout the day as a reminder that God is the central focus of their lives.

### The Ritual Prayer (*Salah*)

In Islam, the five daily prayers (*salah*, sg. /*salawat*, pl.) order a Muslim's day and are a direct connection between the worshipper and God. The ritualized, formalized *salawat* take place from first light to just before dawn (*fajr*), about noon (*dhuhr*), late afternoon (*asr*), just after sunset (*maghrib*), and any time at night (*isha'*). Prayer times, because they are determined by the position of the sun in the sky, change throughout the year. Worldwide prayer times can be found at http://www.islamicity.com/prayerTimes.

Before making *salah*, the Qur'an says that Muslims must perform ritual ablutions (*wudu*) of their hands, faces, and feet.[1] *Salah* is unacceptable without this ablution and without making proper intention (*niyya*) for prayer. Modest clean clothing is required. Men must cover themselves from the navel to the knees. Women must cover entirely, except for their hands, faces, and feet. The movements of the ritualized prayer involve reverently standing, bowing, and prostrating. In mix-gender congregant prayer, women usually pray at the back of the room or in a separate area. This allows them to make the *salah* movements of bowing and prostrating comfortably behind the men. Worshippers need a clean place upon which to prostrate. It is for this reason that most Muslims use prayer carpets for an instantly clean space upon which to pray. Bedridden individuals may pray sitting, standing, or lying down, whichever position is the most comfortable for them. In Qur'an 3:191, God says, "[and] who remember God when they stand, and when they sit, and when they lie down to sleep, and [thus] reflect on the creation of the heavens and the earth..." Muslims pray in the direction (*qibla*) of *Al-Ka'ba* in the Great Mosque in Mecca, Saudi Arabia, which is established in Qur'an 2:144: "We have seen thee [O Prophet] often turn thy face towards heaven [for guidance]: and now We shall indeed make thee turn in prayer in a direction which will fulfill thy desire. Turn, then, thy face towards the Inviolable House of Worship [Great Mosque in Mecca]; and wherever you all may be, turn your faces towards it [in prayer]." Muslim scientists determine the *qibla* of prayer of any given city. The *qibla* for American cities is northeast. Prayer times for the U.S. are listed at http://www.islamicity.com/PrayerTimes/. Muslims also are required to make *salah* at funerals, Friday congregational religious services, eclipses of the sun and moon, and at the three-day celebration called the Feast of Fast Breaking or *'Id al-Fitr*, which comes at the end of the month of Ramadan.[2] Muslims perform extra prayers during Ramadan.

### The Almsgiving (*Zakah*)

The third pillar of Islam is almsgiving or *zakah*. Muslims who have a minimum amount of wealth beyond their needs must pay *zakah* yearly. Because *zakah* is due on all forms of wealth, including business holdings and retirement plans, but also has exemptions, calculating *zakah* can be complicated for some people. Sunnis and Shiites calculate *zakah* somewhat differently. A number of websites provide *zakah* calculators for Sunnis, including http://www.islamicity.com/mosque/zakat/Zakat_calculator.shtml and http://zakatchicago.com/Calculate.aspx. An online source for Shia *zakah* calculation could not be found at the time of this writing. *Zakah* is an obligation, while charity (*sadaqa*), is voluntary. However, Muslims are encouraged to distribute voluntary charity frequently, freely, and discreetly. In Islam, helping those in need is next in importance to the worship of God and is an act of service to God. In practicing *zakah*, Muslims acknowledge that God is the owner of the wealth from which they give alms. Not giving *zakah* is a sin and sullies a person's wealth, according to Islamic law. The distinctions of almsgiving are complex and beyond the scope of this book.

Not obligatory upon Muslims, but encouraged by the Qur'an is voluntary charity (*sadaqah*).

### The Fast (*sawm*)

Ramadan is the ninth month of the Islamic calendar. It is a time for increasing prayer, fasting, performing charity, and doing good deeds. The fast (*sawm*) during the holy month of Ramadan is obligatory upon all Muslims. In Qur'an 2:183, God says, "O you who have attained to faith! Fasting is ordained for you as it was ordained for those before you, so that you might remain conscious of God..." Muslims beyond the age of puberty must fast, except women who are pregnant, in labor, have just given birth, or are in menses. Also excluded are travelers,[3] frail elderly people, and the sick. From first light before dawn until sunset, fasting Muslims refrain from eating, drinking, chewing gum, using tobacco, engaging in marital relations, and having bad behavior. The purpose of fasting is to purify the human ego and to reinforce the human dependence on God. God forgives the sins of Muslims able to fast successfully during the month of Ramadan.

The Islamic calendar follows the lunar calendar[4] and therefore is eleven to twelve days shorter than the solar year.[5] In 2009, for example, the month of Ramadan began August 22 and ended September 20, but in 2010, the holy month began August 11 and ended September 9.

The last ten days of the month of Ramadan, particularly the Night of Power or *Lailatul Qadr*, are special to Muslims. *Lailatul Qadr* is when in 610 C.E. that Angel Gabriel revealed the first words of God (the Qur'an) to Prophet Muhammad. In Qur'an 97:3-5, God says *Lailatul Qadr* "is better than a thousand months: in hosts descend in it the angels, bearing inspiration by their Sustainer's leave; from all [evil] that may happen does it make secure, until the rise of dawn." On this night, which occurs during the last ten days of the month of Ramadan (most likely on an odd numbered night), Muslims chant prayers and recite the Qur'an from sunset to sunrise.

A three-day celebration called the Feast of Fast Breaking or *'Id al-Fitr* starts the first day of *Shawwal*, which is the month that follows Ramadan.

### The Pilgrimage (*Hajj*)

Muslims who are able physically and financially are required to make the pilgrimage (*hajj*) to Mecca, Saudi Arabia, once during their lifetime. The *hajj* lasts five days and occurs during the eighth through the thirteenth days of the last month of the Islamic year, *Zul-Hijjah*. During the pilgrimage, Muslim males wear the ritual two-piece white seamless garment, *ihram*, a symbol of "Islam's unity and egalitarianism."[6] Muslim females wear *ihrams* of various colors that cover the body, except for the face, hands, and feet.

One of the primary rituals of the *hajj* is the seven-time counterclockwise circumambulation of the cube-shaped *Al-Ka'ba*, an ancient symbol of monotheism, at the Great Mosque. Muslims believe that prophets Abraham and Ishmael built the original *Al-Ka'ba* as a house of worship of God.[7] Some say that Prophet Adam first erected *Al-Ka'ba*.

On the tenth day of the month, the *hajj* includes a Feast of Sacrifice or '*Id al-Adha*, which commemorates Prophet Abraham's willingness to sacrifice his son Isma'il in obedience to God. Participating in the *hajj* teaches Muslims about the major events of the life of Prophet Abraham, but, most importantly, it teaches them about putting God first in their lives. God forgives the sins of those successfully completing the *hajj*.

The *hajj* is a lifelong aspiration for many Muslims, and some pilgrims save their pilgrimage clothes to be buried in them.

In 2010, about 2.5 million Muslims made the *hajj* to the holy city of Mecca to follow the journey made by Prophet Muhammad 14 centuries ago.

NOTES

[1] Qur'an 5:6: "O you who have attained to faith! When you are about to pray, wash your face, and your hands and arms up to the elbows, and pass your [wet] hands lightly over your head, and [wash] your feet up to the ankles. And if you are in a state requiring total ablution, purify yourselves. But if you are ill, or are travelling, or have just satisfied a want of nature, or have cohabited with a woman, and can find no water - then take resort to pure dust, passing therewith lightly over your face and your hands."

[2] Frederick Mathewson Denny. *An Introduction to Islam.* 2nd ed., (New York: Macmillan, 1994), 119. For the definition of *'Id al-Fitr*, see the "Glossary."

[3] Aminah Assilmi, in a phone interview on March 2, 2010, said that travelers are excused from fasting if they are 50 miles or more from home, although they would be expected to make up days of fasting once they are no longer traveling. She added that modern-day scholars argue that the number of miles should be increased because of today's modes of rapid transportation. Ancient scholars established the 50-mile guideline based on the number of miles a person could walk in three days. Aminah Assilmi (b. 1945 / d. 2010) was a broadcast journalist and former director of the International Union of Muslim Women.

[4] Each month in the lunar calendar is based on the cycles of the moon. In the Islamic calendar, which is called the *Hijri* calendar, each month begins upon the sighting of the first crescent of a new moon.

[5] The solar calendar is based on solar phases, or said another way, is based on the amount of time the Sun takes to return to the same point.

[6] Denny, 131.

[7] Qur'an 2:127, 130: "And when Abraham and Ishmael were raising the foundations of the Temple, [they prayed:] 'O our Sustainer! Accept Thou this from us: for, verily, Thou alone art all-hearing, all-knowing! .... And who, unless he be weak of mind, would want to abandon Abraham's creed, seeing that We have indeed raised him high in this world, and that, verily, in the life to come he shall be among the righteous?"

CHAPTER 4

# ISLAMIC LAW AND MEDICAL ETHICS

For all practicing Muslims, Islam is a way of life. Its codes of behavior are regulated primarily by the Qur'an and secondly by the *Sunna* (actions and words of Prophet Muhammad). Thirdly, Muslims refer to the *shari'a*, a body of religious norms, including law, ethics, and standards for good behavior and character formation. The literal meaning of *shari'a* is "the path or the road leading to the water," but a deeper meaning is "the ordaining of the Way and its proper subject is God."[1] The ultimate goal of the *shari'a* is to enable Muslims to gain nearness to God by promoting right conduct, obedience, and service to God.[2] Most Muslims know the basic rules of their religion, but turn to their religious leaders (imams) or scholars for complicated or unusual situations. In some cases, Muslims seek only advice and counseling from religious leaders; however, in other cases, they seek an authoritative legal ruling (*fatwa*). Muslim patients and their families often refer to the Qur'an when making decisions about medical care. They also ask their religious leaders (imams) for guidance.

Sunni Muslims, who make up 85 percent of the world's Muslim population, rely on four sources for the *shari'a*. These four sources, ranked in their order of importance, are as follows:

1. The Qur'an
2. Actions and words of Prophet Muhammad (*Sunna*)
3. Consensus (*ijma*) of the Muslims, which is premised on a written report (*hadith*) of the following words of Prophet Muhammad: "My nation cannot agree on an error."[3]
4. Reasoning of the Islamic jurists (*ulama'*) by analogy (*qiyas*) or through new interpretation (*ijtihad*)

Shiite Muslims, who make up about 15 percent of the Muslim population, have a more formal religious hierarchy than Sunnis. Only ordained scholars who derive their authority from the historical Imams can interpret the law.[4] Thus, individual discretion and "imam shopping" is less common with Shiites.

The sources of *shari'a* for Shiism differ slightly from Sunnism.
1. The Qur'an
2. Actions and words of Prophet Muhammad (*Sunna*)
3. Actions and words of the Imams
4. Intellect (*'aql*)

Regardless of the differences between the Sunni and Shia Muslims, all Muslims believe that the Qur'an is the direct word of God and is, therefore, infallible. Consequently, in all of Islam, the indisputable authority is only the Qur'an. Next to the Qur'an, Muslims refer to the *Sunna* for guidelines for daily living. An Islamic scholar writes, "For Muslims, the Prophet Muhammad (pbuh)[5] represents the ideal model of human behavior and multiple Qur'anic injunctions order believers to emulate ... him. Since the Prophet Muhammad (pbuh) represents a life lived totally in accord with the moral/legal code of Islam, he is the normative case as well as the explainer of the code."[6]

Within the *shari'a*, there are five categories of actions and behavior: obligatory acts, recommended acts, permissible acts, offensive acts, and unlawful acts.

1. Obligatory (*fard*) acts, such as fasting and praying five times a day, are required of all Muslims.
2. Recommended (*sunna, mandub, mustahabb, fadila,* or *murghab fihi*) acts are not required, but should be done, such as some prayers.
3. Permissible (*mubah*) acts are religiously neutral, for example, a starving person who has to eat the flesh of a dead animal in order to survive.[7] The eating of carrion is considered *haram*, in Islam.
4. Offensive (*makruh*) acts, such as cigarette smoking, draw diverse opinions among Islamic jurists.
5. Unlawful (*haram*) acts are strictly forbidden and include adultery, eating pig meat, and drinking alcoholic beverages.

Categorizing actions is as much a matter of ethics as it is of law. Islamic ethical reasoning employs many "tools" to apply to a particular case. Among these tools are the five legal maxims, "which embody the spirit of [the Islamic] religion,"[8] and are agreed upon as central to all Muslims. These maxims are: "matters will be judged by their purposes; certainty will not be overturned by doubt; harm must be removed; hardship must be alleviated; and custom has the weight of law."[9] An example of a maxim at work is as follows: A forbidden action is not forbidden if the only other possible course of action is more harmful than the first. Eating pork, for instance, is prohibited; however, if pork is the only food available and a person would starve by not eating it, then consuming pork would be permissible.

Moreover, because the "*Sunnah* [sic] is not just a mere catalog of moral behavior; it is a collection of data that requires assessment and application,"[10] Muslims turn to Islamic jurists for moral judgments. These jurists use the primary sources of the Qur'an and *Sunna* as the foundation of their religious opinions (*fatwas*). They also draw upon the third and fourth sources of Islamic law – consensus (*ijma*) and analogical deduction (*qiyas*). The precedent for this process of rendering *fatwas* comes from the following. In this report, Prophet Muhammad gave judge Mu'adh ibn Jabal tacit approval to issue religious opinions.

> The Prophet asks, 'How will you decide when a question arises?' He replied: 'According to the Book of Allah.' 'And if you do not find the answer in the Book of Allah?' 'Then according to the sunna of the Messenger of Allah.' 'And if you do not find the answer neither in the sunna nor in the Book?' 'Then I shall come to a decision according to my own opinion without hesitation.' Then the Messenger of Allah slapped Mu'adh on the chest with his hand saying: 'Praise be to Allah who has led the messenger of the Messenger of Allah to an answer that pleased him.'"[11]

Today's advances in medical science (e.g., stem cell research) are prompting bioethical dilemmas among Muslims. In such cases, Muslims turn to Islamic jurists' religious rulings (*fatwas*). The jurists "analyze every question in light of the principles laid down by the Qur'an and Sunna as well as in the light of the standards set by earlier jurists enumerated in the books of Islamic jurisprudence. This exercise is known as *istinbat* or *ijtihad*... [and it is] the ongoing process of *istinbat* [that] keeps injecting new ideas, concepts and rulings into the heritage of Islamic jurisprudence."[12]

NOTES

1. Fazlur Rahman, *Major Themes of the Qur'an* (Minneapolis, Minnesota: Bibliotheca Islamica, 1989), 100.

2 Aasim I. Padela, "Islamic Medical Ethics: A Primer," *Bioethics* 21, No. 3 (2007): 174.

3 Ibid.

4 *Ithna 'Ashariyya* believe there are only twelve rightly guided Imams; the Ismaili Shia hold to seven, and the Zaydi Shia embrace five. These historical leaders are the direct descendants of the Prophet Muhammad and according to Shia belief, are able to guide today's believers.

5 The acronym "pbuh" means "peace and blessing of Allah be upon him." This phrase is said after saying the name of a prophet, as encouraged by Qur'an 33:56 and *ahadith* (reports of the words and actions of the Prophet Muhammad). The phrase is shortened to "pbuh" in documents.

6 Padela, 175.

7 Yahya ibn Sharaf al-Nawawi, *Al-Maqasid, Nawawi's Manual of Islam*, trans. Nuh Ha Mim Keller (Beltsville, MD: Amana Publications, 2002), 8-9.

[8] Umar Faruq Abd-Allah, “Living Islam with Purpose” (Nawawi Foundation Paper, 2007), 3, http://www.nawawi.org/downloads/article6.pdf. Accessed 20 November 2009.

[9] Ibid.

[10] Padela, 175.

[11] M.Th. Houtsma, *E.J. Brill’s First Encyclopaedia of Islam, 1913-1936*, Vol. 5 (Leiden, Netherlands: E.J. Brill, 1993), 1052.

[12] Mahmoud A. el-Gamal, *Islamic Finance: Law, Economics, and Practice* (New York: Cambridge University Press, 2006), 17, quoting M.T. Usmani, *An Introduction to Islamic Finance* (Karachi: Idaratul Ma’arif, 1998), 237.

CHAPTER 5

# ISLAMIC RELIGIOUS AUTHORITY

As previously noted, the theological difference between the two branches of Islam, Shiism and Sunnism, stems from disagreement about who should succeed Prophet Muhammad (d. 632 C.E.). In the seventh century, some believed that 'Ali ibn Abu Talib, cousin and son-in-law of Prophet Muhammad, was the rightful successor. Eventually, 'Ali ibn Abu Talib became the fourth *caliph*, but he was murdered in 661 C.E. in a mosque in Kufa (near Najaf, Iraq). His son and successor, Husayn ibn 'Ali, followed him in death, when he, along with seventy-two followers and family members, were massacred on the Plain of Karbala (southern Iraq) in 680 C.E.

The death of Husayn galvanized his followers, who later became known as the Shiites ("Group" or "Sect"). Devotion to 'Ali ibn Abu Talib is at the heart of Shiism. About 80 percent or 150 million of today's Shiites are Twelver-Imam (*Ithna 'ashariyya*). They believe in the divinely ordained authority of their first Imam,[1] 'Ali ibn Abu Talib, and in the eleven divinely appointed *Imami* successors (*Khalifa Ilahi*). These eleven Imams were the direct descendants of Prophet Muhammad and 'Ali ibn Abu Talib. Shiites believe that these Imams also inherited special religious authority from Prophet Muhammad and 'Ali ibn Abu Talib. Along with political power, the Shiites ascribed infallibility to the Imams' interpretations of the Qur'an. After the disappearance of the twelfth Imam, Muhammad al Madhi, in the tenth century, there arose imams and *ayatollahs* (signs of God) who believed in the authority of the Imams and who upheld their traditions. These men hold both political and religious power. Their followers believe that their interpretations of the Qur'an and God's will are absolute. The *ayatollahs* are the leaders of today's Shia community.

The Twelver-Imam has only one school of jurisprudence, the Jafari School. Jafari jurists use the Qur'an as the primary source and the reports of the actions and words of Prophet Muhammad (*hadith*, sg. / *ahadith*, pl.) as the secondary source; however, they also refer to the *ahadith* of the Twelve Imams.

The other two branches of Shiism are the Ismaili and the Zaydi, which, respectively, ascribe to seven and five divinely ordained Imams. Both have their own schools of religious law.

Most Shiites reside in Azerbaijan, Bahrain, Iran, Iraq, and Oman, with large populations in India, Lebanon, Pakistan, Syria, and Yemen.

In contrast, Sunnis do not assign divine guidance or appointment to the religious leaders (imams). Sunnis believe that the most qualified person should lead the community and that only Prophet Muhammad was able to interpret the Qur'an and the will of God without error. All Sunni Muslim legal scholars (*ulama*) interpret the Qur'an and the Sunna (actions and words of Prophet Muhammad) in rendering their interpretative religious law, but they have many different legal and theological schools and allow for diversity of interpretation in their community. Most Sunnis belong to one of four schools of religious law (*madhhab*): Hanafi, Hanbali, Maliki, and Shafi'i. The schools differ in the way they balance various scriptural passages, reason, custom, and authority. Some Muslims do not identify with a school; these include "*salafi*" Muslims who try to interpret from scripture directly and attempt to follow the literal meaning of the Qur'an and the *Sunna*, as well as the modernists, who emphasize the context of an overall ethical message of revelation more than the literal meaning of revelation.

Among the followers of the schools of religious law, the cords of the 1,400-year-old faith tradition of Islam unite Shiite and Sunni Muslims, although minor variances of worship practices do exist. For example, with regard to the obligatory daily prayers (*salah*), Shia Muslims may combine the noon (*dhur*) and afternoon prayers (*asr*) and also the after sunset (*maghrib*) and night prayers (*isha*'). On the other hand, Sunnis pray each prayer separately, but can combine prayers under specific conditions.

Issues of gender and religious authority are controversial among most world religions. In Islam, Muslim men dominate as religious scholars and religious leaders (imams). Muslim women, according to traditional interpretations of Islam, may not lead prayer or preach in mixed-gender congregations. Muslim traditionalists contend that the Qur'an allows only men to do both. They cite the following *hadith*: "The best rows for men are the first rows, and the worst ones the last ones, and the best rows for women are the last ones and the worst ones for them are the first ones."[2] Others say that the Qur'an specifically does not prohibit women from leading prayer or preaching in mixed-gender congregations. They point to a *hadith* about a woman named Umm Waraqa, whom Prophet Muhammad allowed to lead prayer in her male/female household.[3] Additionally, some scholars say that women may lead prayer and preach, but only to other women. In China, Muslim women serve as imams to other women.[4]

Nevertheless, today's Muslim women are asserting themselves as religious authorities and are teaching and interpreting Islam. They are influential forces at home, in the mosques, and in their communities. The issue of gender equality is of utmost importance in Islam and has been since the beginning of the religion in the seventh century. A basic principle of Islam – the equality of humankind, regardless of gender – comes from the Qur'an. In Qur'an 33:35, God says that women are equals to men and that men and women share equal responsibilities and rewards.

> Verily, for all men and women who have surrendered themselves unto God, and all believing men and believing women, and all truly devout men and truly devout women, and all men and women who are true to their word, and all men and women who are patient in adversity, and all men and women who humble themselves [before God], and all men and women who give in charity, and all self-denying men and self-denying women, and all men and women who are mindful of their chastity, and all men and women who remember God unceasingly: for [all of] them has God readied forgiveness of sins and a mighty reward.

NOTES

[1] English translations capitalize "Imams" when referring to the first twelve Shia religious leaders. Sunnis do not capitalize "imams" when referring to their religious leaders.

[2] Muslim ibn al-Hajjaj, *Sahih Muslim*, Book 4, Number 881, University of Southern California *ahadith* database: http://www.usc.edu/schools/college/crcc/engagement/resources/texts/muslim/hadith/muslim/004.smt.html. Accessed 2 April 2010.

[3] "The Messenger of Allah used to visit her [Umm Waraqa] in her house. And he assigned to her a *muadhdhin* who would make the summons to prayer (*adhan*) for her. And he asked her to lead the inhabitants of her home." This *hadith* is attributed to Sunan Abu Dawood in an article entitled "Real Debate about the Status of Women" by Aslam Abdullah that appeared on the website of Islamicity.com, http://www.islamicity.com/articles/Articles.asp?ref=IC0503-2643. Accessed 3 April 2010. Umm Waraqa also cared for the wounded men on the battlefield. Umar, the second caliph, appointed Umm Waraqa to lead the large market committees of Medina and Mecca.

[4] Vali Nasr and Seyyed Vali Reza Nasr, *Forces of Fortune: The Rise of the New Muslim Middle Class and What It Will Mean for Our World* (New York: Free Press, 2009), 189.

## CHAPTER 6

# HEALTHCARE SENSITIVITIES AND RELATED ISSUES

The moral code of Islam is derived from the Qur'an, the words and deeds (*Sunna*) of Prophet Muhammad, and the religious opinions (*fatwas*) of Islamic jurists. Together, they create a religious culture for Muslims. The many ethnicities of Muslims also influence the religious culture. Healthcare sensitivities and related issues formed by these sources affect dietary regulations, fasting, gender modesty, and women's rights, among other issues.

### Dietary Regulations

1. The dietary regulations of Islam promote the health and well-being of Muslims. These regulations "are a means of sanctifying everyday life"[1] and are based in the Qur'an, the primary source of Islamic law, as exemplified by the life, actions, and teachings of Prophet Muhammad (*Sunna*), the secondary source of Islamic law.

2. Muslims are mandated to follow the Islamic dietary laws whether traveling or during illness (where possible).

3. Only foods and liquids expressly prohibited (*haram*) by the Qur'an and *Sunna* are off-limits to Muslims. Qur'an 2:173: "He [God] has forbidden to you only carrion, and blood, and the flesh of swine, and that over which any name other than God's has been invoked; but if one is driven by necessity neither coveting it nor exceeding his immediate need no sin

shall be upon him: for, behold, God is much-forgiving, a dispenser of grace."

4. Qur'an 5:3 says:

> Forbidden to you is carrion, and blood, and the flesh of swine, and that over which any name other than God's has been invoked, and the animal that has been strangled, or beaten to death, or killed by a fall, or gored to death, or savaged by a beast of prey, save that which you [yourselves] may have slaughtered while it was still alive; and [forbidden to you is] all that has been slaughtered on idolatrous altars.

5. Muslims are prohibited from eating pork, blood, carrion, carnivores, and birds of prey.

6. Qur'an 6:118 says: "So eat of (meats) on which Allah's name hath been pronounced, if ye have faith in His Signs." The various Islamic schools of religious thought interpret this verse differently. The "Hanafi school, taking these words at their face value prohibits all meat upon which the name of God has not been recited. The Shafi'i school, however, followed by the Hanbali and Maliki schools (the Shi'a hold the position similar to the Hanafi), hold that this prohibition cannot be accepted at face value. They argue that basically what has been prohibited is the meat of an animal that has been offered to any other being except God ..."[2] Scholars of these schools historically contextualize the Qur'anic injunction, saying that in the early years of Islam, those butchers in Mecca who converted to Islam "were suspected by Muslims of mentioning their erstwhile gods' names 'in their hearts' while slaughtering animals."[3] Today, therefore "in a situation where there was no such suspicion it was

not thought necessary to recite God's name. The adoption of this liberal interpretation enables many Muslims to buy meat prepared by Non-Muslim butchers…"[4]

7. Muslims are prohibited from consuming alcohol. Islamic scholars' and jurists' religious rulings (*fatwas*) forbidding the usage of intoxicants are based on Qur'an 5:90-91. In it, God says, "O You who have attained to faith! Intoxicants, and games of chance, and idolatrous practices, and the divining of the future are but a loathsome evil of Satan's doing: shun it, then, so that you might attain to a happy state! By means of intoxicants and games of chance Satan seeks only to sow enmity and hatred among you, and to turn you away from the remembrance of God and from prayer. Will you not, then, desist?"

8. Unless there are no alternatives, Muslims may refuse healthcare products (insulin, for example, or some homeopathic remedies) that contain pig or alcohol or any *haram* items mentioned above, including capsulated medicines made from pig gelatin. Those Muslims ascribing to the Hanafi School of religious thought, however, are permitted alcohol for medical purposes.[5]

9. Islamic law permits (*halal*) all other foods and liquids. In Qur'an 2:172, God says: "O you who have attained to faith! Partake of the good things which We have provided for you as sustenance, and render thanks unto God, if it is [truly] Him that you worship."

10. Depending on a Muslim's particular religious school of law, he/she may eat lawful (*halal*) fish with scales, shrimp, or all seafood. Muslims may eat herbivore animals, but these animals must be ritually slaughtered according to Islamic guidelines.

11. However, herbivore game animals that Muslims hunted or fished do not have to be ritually slaughtered, because Islam considers game animals ritually pure.
12. All grains, fruits, legumes, and vegetables may be eaten.
13. Most Kosher-sanctioned food products are permissible, but are not interchangeable with *halal.*
14. Information about the Islamic dietary regulations is available at http://www.islamicity.com/food; and at http://www.muslimconsumer-group.com/General.do;jsessionid=52567A6E267ACE3BFA45D06C2AABAE2D?menu=Home&eventAction=init. Another source is *Halal food production* by Mian N. Riaz and Muhammad M. Chaudry, published in 2004 by CRC Press, Boca Raton, Florida.

### Fasting (*sawm*)

1. Muslims worldwide observe the holy month of Ramadan, which is the ninth month of the year. During this month, from before sunrise to after sunset, Muslims are required to fast (*sawm*) from drinking liquids, eating, using tobacco products, and intimate relations.
2. Anything liquid or solid taken in through any orifice breaks the fast.
3. There are exemptions to *sawm*, however. Sick people are not required to fast, but may choose to do so, unless harmful to their health.[6]
4. Other Muslims excused from fasting are elderly frail people, menstruating and pregnant women, those traveling more than fifty miles from home, children under the age of puberty (although they are encouraged to "practice" fasting to the extent they are able), and individuals with learning challenges or developmental delays.

## Gender Modesty

1. Some Muslim men and women may want to be cared for by the same-gender healthcare providers (physicians, nurses, etc.), and then some only if a family member is present. The Qur'an and *ahadith* (reports of the words and deeds of Prophet Muhammad) literature speak of gender modesty. Qur'an 24:30-31 says:

> Tell the believing men to lower their gaze and to be mindful of their chastity: this will be most conducive to their purity – [and,] verily, God is aware of all that they do. And tell the believing women to lower their gaze and to be mindful of their chastity, and not to display their charms [in public] beyond what may [decently] be apparent thereof…

2. However, there is *hadith* precedent for opposite-gender care when a same-gender provider is unavailable. One *hadith*, in particular, reports about women caring for wounded men on the battlefield. "We used to take part in holy battles with the Prophet [Muhammad] by providing the people with water and serving them and bringing the killed and the wounded back to Medina."[8] Yet, *hadith* states that "the Medinese woman Umm 'Atiya, a nurse and companion of the Prophet, reports, 'I accompanied the Prophet in seven battles. I rode behind men in their saddles; I used to prepare food for them, treat the wounded and the sick.'"[9]

3. Despite modesty, the "necessity of saving a life supersedes all dictates of modesty and care. During resuscitations or other emergent procedures, any available healthcare provider may examine and perform procedures on a Muslim patient."[10]

4. In particular, Muslim women have difficulty with male hospital employees, clinicians, or others entering their rooms without first announcing themselves. Out of respect for the modesty of female Muslim patients, the hospital staff should establish some sort of signal that would give female patients ample time to cover themselves.
5. If a Muslim woman shares a room with a patient who has visiting male relatives and friends, the two patients should agree to have the curtain drawn around the bed of the Muslim patient in order to protect her privacy and modesty.

## Ritual Prayer (*Salah*)

1. God revealed the ritual prayer (*salah*) to Prophet Muhammad. *Salah* is the second of five required worship practices (pillars) of Islam.
2. All Muslims, from the age of puberty to the time of death, are obligated to perform *salah* five times daily, every day. Only those too ill or women in their menses are excused from *salah*. Sick people are permitted to pray as they are able, whether sitting, lying down, or standing, and with or without ablutions, and with or without wearing clean clothing. *Salah* is performed from first light to just before dawn (*fajr*), about noon (*dhuhr*), late afternoon (*asr*), just after sunset (*maghrib*), and any time at night (*isha'*). For prayer times by location worldwide, go to http://www.islamicity.com/prayerTimes/.
3. Using clean running water, Muslims must make ritual ablutions (*wudu*) of their hands, faces, arms, feet, and the top of their heads before *salah*.
4. Muslim men must wear clean clothes that cover from their waists to

their feet. Muslim women must clean clothes that cover their bodies: head (not including the face for most Muslims), arms, torso, and legs to the ankles.

5. Muslims stand on prayer rugs (for cleanliness), turn toward the *qibla* of *Al-Ka'ba* in the Great Mosque in Mecca, Saudi Arabia, and set their intention (*niyya*) to do *salah*. *Qibla* means the "direction" of *Al-Ka'ba*, which is the house of worship built by prophets Abraham and Ishmael. Some Muslims believe that Prophet Adam first erected *Al-Ka'ba*.

6. *Salah* involves recitation of Qur'an and standing, sitting, kneeling, and prostrating.

7. *Salah* may take up to 20 minutes, but usually takes less time. Healthcare providers should be sensitive to prayer times. A signal should be agreed upon between the patient and her/his attending nurse to alert others wanting to enter the room that the patient is doing *salah*, and to wait. For example, if while a Muslim patient is praying there is a knock on the door of the room, that patient could clap to signal that he/she is in prayer. Another means would be to place a sign on the door.

8. Speaking during *salah* invalidates the prayer.

9. Walking in front of a Muslim making *salah* is disrespectful.

### Ritual Purity

1. Most Muslims use only the right hand for eating, drinking, and shaking hands, and the left hand for cleaning themselves after using the toilet.

2. On the Day of Judgment, those receiving their book of deeds in their left hands go to Hell, and those receiving their book of deeds in their right hands go to Heaven.

3. Ritual purity is required before making the five-times daily prayer (*salah*), and before touching and reciting the Qur'an.
4. Sexual intercourse, ejaculation, menstruation, flatulence, urinating, defecating, vomiting, falling asleep, fainting or passing out, and intoxication break ritual purity. The flow of blood or pus or other fluids from the body also breaks ritual purity.
5. The individual ritual purity practices are *ghusl*, *istinja*, *tayammum*, and *wudu*.
6. *Ghusl* is an Arabic word that means "bathing;" however, for convenience, Muslims often do *ghusl* in the shower. *Ghusl* is a stepped process that involves using clean, running water to purify the body. It is required after sexual intercourse, ejaculation, at the end of monthly menstruation, and at the end of the confinement period of women after childbirth (up to 40 days). *Ghusl* also is performed on the body of a deceased person.
7. *Istinja* literally means "to remove harmful things." This form of ritual ablution is done after urinating or defecating, and involves using water to clean the anus and genitals. The Prophet Muhammad excused sick people from doing *istinja*. He "insisted that those entitled to be excused from any such duty carried no blame, and he would grow angry with sick people, who out of misplaced piety performed ablution rites which might endanger their health."[11] Muslims too sick to make *istinja* may still perform *salah*.
8. *Tayammum* or dry ablution may be made by Muslims too sick to complete *wudu*, or for others when there is not enough clean water. *Tayammum* involves touching a stone or clean dust with both hands and moving the hands over the face, hands and forearms. "The Prophet

Muhammad said in reference to a companion who had a wound to his head. The companions gave him advice that he must do a complete ablution. The Prophet said it would have been enough for him to do *tayammum* because he died as a result of the ablution and the wounded head."[12]

9. *Wudu* is the action of washing with clean water, preferably using running water, the mouth, nostrils, face, hands, and forearms, and wiping the head and ears, and washing the feet.

### Predestination, Sickness, and Trauma

1. Cultural and religious beliefs influence each Muslim's understanding of disease and health. For example, some believe in predestination and maintain that sickness and trauma come from God. Thus, they do not believe in accepting medical treatment for illness or injury.

2. Other Muslims adhere to the teaching that they must do everything possible to maintain their health, and to save their lives and the lives of others.

### The Qur'an

1. Muslims believe that the Qur'an is absolutely the infallible and actual words of God as revealed in the language of Arabic 1,400 years ago to Prophet Muhammad by Angel Gabriel.[13] The original Qur'an compiled into book-form in the 650s C.E. is the same today as it was fourteen centuries ago. The Qur'anic manuscript is called *mushaf* (pronounced *mus-haf*). Muslims believe that a translation is only an interpretation of the Qur'an.

2. Most Muslim patients want a Qur'an at the bedside. They maintain a state of ritual purification when touching the Qur'an.
3. Non-Muslims should handle the Qur'an respectfully. Ask permission before moving a Qur'an, and when doing so, make sure not to place the holy book on the floor or under other books or items.

## HEALTHCARE DECISIONS

1. Most Muslim patients want to know what is going on with their health. They want to make their own choices.
2. A few or some Muslim patients, however, may want clinicians to discuss healthcare issues with their family members; however, for hospital records, these patients must inform the appropriate healthcare personnel of their preference.
3. Married couples frequently make healthcare decisions together.
4. Unmarried patients look to their closest relatives for determining the best course of treatment. They may rely on their relatives to convey that information to clinicians.
5. Provide the patient care bill of rights to teenage patients. Some parents may not want to involve their teenage children in healthcare discussions. Use your judgement, but always put concern for the teenage patient first.

## NON-MUSLIM VISITATION

1. Upon meeting Muslim patients, be mindful that most Muslims do not shake hands with people of the opposite gender.
2. Shaking hands or any form of physical contact with members of the opposite gender is reserved only for spouses and immediate family members.

3. The basis for moral conduct in Islam comes primarily from the Qur'an and then from the words and actions of Prophet Muhammad (*Sunna*). A report (*hadith*) of Prophet Muhammad says that when he accepted oaths of allegiance from female Muslim converts, "he never touched the hand of any women (i.e. never shook hands with them) while taking the pledge of allegiance and he never took their pledge of allegiance except by his words (only)."[14]

4. As a form of greeting, some Muslims may touch their right hand to their heart.

5. Many Muslims may avoid prolonged eye contact with people of the opposite gender who are not part of their family. This practice of gender modesty or respect stems from Qur'an 24:30-31: "Tell the believing men to lower their gaze and to be mindful of their chastity: this will be most conducive to their purity – [and,] verily, God is aware of all that they do. And tell the believing women to lower their gaze and to be mindful of their chastity, and not to display their charms [in public] ..." As such, avoid making prolonged eye contact with Muslim patients of the opposite gender.

6. The following suggestions for greeting Muslim patients, family members or friends may be helpful.

- Announce yourself before entering the room of a female Muslim patient in order to give her time to cover or put on a headscarf (*hijab*). Afford the same respect to a male Muslim patient.
- Offer the greeting of *assalamu 'alaykum* (peace be unto you).

9. If the patient first offers the greeting of *assalamu 'alaykum*, respond with *wa 'alaykum assalam* (and peace be unto you).

- Leave the patient's door ajar or curtain partially open when visiting a patient of the opposite gender.

### IMAMS

1. Sunni Islam has no clergy. It has imams (those who stand in front). Sunni imams are adult males, are not ordained, hold only limited religious authority, and are often self-taught, but some hold academic degrees in theology. Sunni imams are community-appointed.
2. To become an imam, a Muslim must have sufficient knowledge of the Qur'an and the words and actions of Prophet Muhammad (*Sunna*), the primary sources of Islamic law (*shari'a*), to be qualified to lead prayers at mosques, deliver the sermon (*khutba*) at Friday prayer (*Jum'ah*) at a mosque, perform marriages, and preside at funerals.
3. In the absence of an imam, any mature male Muslim knowledgeable in Islam may lead prayers and perform marital or burial rituals.
4. Muslims turn to imams with questions and concerns about the *shari'a* and other Islamic-related issues.
5. Some culturally oriented and first-generation immigrant imams, because of having little to no exposure to the American culture and because of being able to speak only their native languages, may be more of an obstacle than a help when working with healthcare providers on behalf of Muslim patients, even though these imams are overwhelmingly qualified in Islam.

### VISITATION OF THE SICK AND DYING

1. There is much evidence in the *hadith* literature that Prophet

Muhammad encouraged Muslims to visit the sick and the dying. One such report from Abu Huraira, a companion of Prophet Muhammad, is as follows:

> God shall say on the Day of Judgment, 'O son of Adam! I was sick but you did not visit me.' 'My Lord! How could I visit you when you are the Lord of the whole world,' man will reply. God will say, 'Did you not know that so and so from among my servants [that is, human beings] was sick but you never visited him or her? Did you not know that if you had visited, you would have found me there? O son of Adam! I was hungry but you did not feed me?' 'How could I feed you Lord! When you are the Lord of the world?' God shall answer, 'Did you not know that so and so of my servants was hungry and asked you for food, but you did not feed him or her. Did you not know that if you had given food you would have found requital here?'[15]

2. Expect family members to visit their hospitalized loved one, to bring ethnic foods, and to pray with them. The traditional Muslim family often includes three or more generations, and most likely, all of them will be present when their loved one is dying. In Islam, family is "regarded as the cornerstone of a healthy and balanced society."[16]
3. Additionally, Muslims are exhorted by Prophet Muhammad to be of good cheer in the presence of patients. "People visiting the sick are asked to say such things to them as would make them [patients] happy…"[17]
4. Prophet Muhammad "encouraged visitors to request the sick person to pray for them because the state of the sick and the helpless is so pure that God hears their prayers."[18]

## Women's Rights

1. Procreation is one of the main objectives of marriage. Therefore, mutual spousal consent is required for procreation, birth control, and for procedures that prevent procreation. In Islam, only heterosexual couples are permitted to marry and have children.
2. Women have the right to inherit, own property, accumulate wealth, choose their religion and husband, and pursue education and career. Islam affirms these rights, but some Muslims follow their cultural practices, which might deny women these rights. In such cases, an authoritative religious opinion is helpful.
3. Qur'an 33:35 says that women are equal to men in the eyes of God and that men and women share equal responsibilities and rewards.

## Domestic Violence

1. Treatment of women is as diverse as the Muslim countries and communities themselves.
2. Domestic violence knows no boundaries. Worldwide, it is the leading cause of death among women ages 14 to 44.[19] In America, "one in every four women will experience domestic violence in her lifetime."[20] It is estimated that about 10 percent of Muslim women suffer from domestic violence.[21]
3. Domestic abuse stems from false justifications or tribal or cultural traditions of Muslims in nearly every country. It is the extreme of the intolerable discrimination and oppression of women of any age, economic status, race, religion, nationality, or educational background.
4. Domestic violence violates the Qur'anic principle of gender equality.

> Quran 33:35 says: Verily, for all men and women who have surrendered themselves unto God, and all believing men and believing women, and all truly devout men and truly devout women, and all men and women who are true to their word, and all men and women who are patient in adversity, and all men and women who humble themselves [before God], and all men and women who give in charity, and all self-denying men and self-denying women, and all men and women who are mindful of their chastity, and all men and women who remember God unceasingly: for [all of] them has God readied forgiveness of sins and a mighty reward.

5. Domestic abuse violates the message of peace of Islam. Qur'an 30:21 says, "And among His wonders is this: He creates for you mates out of your own kind, so that you might incline towards them, and He engenders love and tenderness between you: in this, behold, there are messages indeed for people who think!"
6. Those who perpetrate violence upon women often refer to Qur'an 4:34:

> Men shall take full care of women with the bounties which God has bestowed more abundantly on the former than on the latter, and with what they may spend out of their possessions. And the righteous women are the truly devout ones, who guard the intimacy which God has [ordained to be] guarded. And as for those women whose ill-will you have reason to fear, admonish them [first]; then leave them alone in bed; then beat them; and if thereupon they pay you heed, do not seek to harm them. Behold, God is indeed most high, great!

7. According to Islamic scholar Jamal Badawi, Muslims are not permitted "to cause any bodily harm or even be harsh." The "beating" referred to in the above translation of the Qur'an, he says, was interpreted by early Islamic jurists as "light striking … as a (symbolic) use or *miswak* (a small natural toothbrush)."[22]

8. A report of Prophet Muhammad (*hadith*) says, "I went to the Apostle of Allah (peace be upon him) and asked him: 'What do you say (command) about our wives?' He replied: 'Give them food what you have for yourself, and clothe them by which you clothe yourself, and do not beat them, and do not revile them.'"[23]

9. The bottom line is this: The abuse of women is a domestic violence issue. It is not intrinsic to the faith tradition of Islam.

---

NOTES

[1] Vali Nasr and Seyyed Vali Reza Nasr, *Forces of Fortune: The Rise of the New Muslim Middle Class and What It Will Mean for Our World* (New York: Free Press, 2009), 128.

[2] Fazlur Rahman, *Health and Medicine in the Islamic Tradition*, (New York: Crossroad Publishing, 1989), 54.

[3] Ibid.

[4] Ibid.

[5] Ibid.

[6] Kamyar M. Hedayat and Raya Pirzedeh, "Issues in Islamic Biomedical Ethics: A Primer for the Pediatrician," *Pediatrics* 108, No. 4 (October 2001): 970; citing Sane'i Y, *Istifaa'al-e Pezeshky* (Qom, Iran: Maithan Tamat Publications: 1998) 207. Ruling No. 629.

[8] Muhammad ibn Ismail al-Bukhari, *Sahih Bukhari,* Volume 4, Book 52, Number 134, University of Southern California *ahadith* database: http://www.usc.edu/schools/college/crcc/engagement/resources/texts/muslim/hadith/bukhari/052.sbt.html. Accessed 4 April 2010.

[9] Rahman, 55.

[10] Hedayat and Pirzedeh, ibid.

[11] Tim J. Winter, "The Muslim grand narrative," in *Caring for Muslim Patients,* 2nd ed. Eds. Aziz Sheikh and Abdul Rashid Gatrad, (Oxon, United Kingdom: Radcliffe Publishing, 2009), 28.

[12] The *hadith* comes from Mohamed Magid, executive director of the All Dulles Area Muslim Society (ADAMS) in Washington, D.C., and president of the Islamic Society of North America, in an email dated March 4, 2010. Imam Magid attributed this saying of the Prophet Muhammad to "Imam Abu Dawud and Al-Munduri."

[13] N.J. Dawood, trans., *The Koran* (New York: Penguin Books, 1986), 9. Dawood, in the introductory comments of his translation, wrote that excepting "only the opening verses and some few passages in which the Prophet Muhammad or the Angel Gabriel speak in the first person, the speaker throughout [the Qur'an] is God."

[14] Muhammad ibn Ismail al-Bukhari, *Sahih Bukhari,* Volume 3, Book 50, Number 874, from the University of Southern California *ahadith* database: http://www.usc.edu/schools/college/crcc/engagement/resources/texts/muslim/hadith/bukhari/050.sbt.html, Accessed 17 April 2010.

[15] Rahman, 59.

[16] Sangeeta Dhami and Aziz Sheikh, "The family: predicament and promise," in *Caring for Muslim Patients,* 57.

[17] Rahman, 59.

[18] Ibid.

[19] National Organization for Women, "NOW Supports Legislation that Denounces 'Honor' Killings and Violence Against Women," http://www.now.org/press/10-07/10-08b.html. Accessed 4 April 2010.

[20] The National Domestic *The New York Times Almanac 2002.* New York: Penguin, 2001.

[21] Kamran Memon, "Wife Abuse in the Muslim Community," http://www.themodernreligion.com/women/w_abuse1.htm#comm. Accessed 4 April 2010.

[22] Jamal Badwai, "Is wife beating allowed in Islam?" http://www.themodernreligion.com/women/w_abuse_badawi.htm. Accessed 4 April 2010.

[23] Abu Dawud, *Sunan Abu-Dawud,* Book 11, Number 2139, University of Southern California *ahadith* database: http://www.usc.edu/schools/college/crcc/engagement/resources/texts/muslim/hadith/abudawud/011.sat.html. Accessed 4 April 2010.

## CHAPTER 7

# ABORTION

Ahmed and Hamda are excitedly expecting their second child, a girl. They already have named her Amina, but their excitement is dashed after a routine ultrasound turns up what doctors suspect to be a birth defect. More sophisticated testing confirms a hole in the diaphragm of the 17-week-old baby, a condition known as congenital diaphragmatic hernia (CDH). In baby Amina's case, her stomach, intestines, liver and spleen had migrated from the abdomen into the chest cavity and are preventing the development of the left lung.

One in every 2,500 babies suffers from CDH, and about half die. Some parents opt for abortion. For Ahmed and Hamda, both devout Muslims, abortion is out of the question. They want to save the baby. Physicians tell them that moving the organs to the abdomen and repairing the diaphragmatic hernia would put the mother and baby at fatal risk. They also tell Hamda that if she carries the baby to term, she could die. The couple prays for guidance and consults with their imam (religious leader) before deciding to terminate the pregnancy.

### Islamic Perspective on Abortion

In Islam, although abortion is permitted under certain circumstances, which may vary by religious legal school, the majority of scholars insist that a Muslim woman cannot simply decide to end a pregnancy without cause. This type of reproductive freedom does not exist in Islam, because the sanctity of life – including that of a fetus – is an injunction. In Qur'an 4:29, God says, "... do not destroy one another: for, behold, God is indeed a dispenser of grace unto you!" In Qur'an 4:93, the Creator says, "... whoever deliberately slays another believer, his requital shall be hell, therein to abide; and God will condemn him, and will reject him, and will prepare for him awesome suffering."

Islamic law (*shari'a*) does not specifically mention abortion (*saqt*), but Islamic jurists (*fuqaha'*) have rendered a number of legal assessments (*fatwas*) on the subject. Sunni scholar Yusuf Qaradawi writes that abortion "constitutes an offense against a complete, living human being."[1] Qaradawi and most Islamic Sunni jurists, however, do permit abortion, but only before fetal ensoulment (see below), and only if continuing the pregnancy jeopardizes the mother's life or in cases of severe fetal deformity. Shia cleric Shaykh Ali Sistani[2] does not permit abortions once the zygote (the cell that results from fertilization) has implanted itself in the womb. Some jurists also allow abortions of severely deformed fetuses among other situations (see below).

### What is Ensoulment?

Ensoulment (also called personhood) occurs when the spirit (*ruh*) enters the fetus. Qur'an 32:6-9 says, " ...the Almighty, the Dispenser of Grace ... begins the creation of [the human] out of clay; then He causes [the human] to be begotten out of the essence of a humble fluid; and then He forms [the human] in accordance with what [the human] is meant to be, and breathes into [the human] of His spirit ..." Jurists have mixed opinions about when the *ruh* enters the fetus. Some say it occurs 40 days after conception and others conclude that it is 120 days, based on Qur'an 23:12-14, which describes the five stages of the first 120 days of intrauterine life: from sperm to "germ-cell" to "embryonic lump" to the formation of bones and then "We clothe the bones with flesh..." The following *hadith* breaks down the five stages into increments of 40 days. In it, Prophet Muhammad said,

> ...every one of you is collected in the womb of his mother for the first forty days, and then he becomes a clot for another forty days, and then a piece of flesh for another forty days. Then Allah sends an angel to write four words: He writes his deeds, time of his death, means of his livelihood, and whether he will be wretched or blessed (in religion). Then the soul is breathed into his body.[3]

When the soul is breathed in the body, it is at this point that the fetus "becomes a 'real person.'"[4]

The Islamic jurists of the four major Sunni schools of jurisprudence, Hanafi, Hanbali, Maliki, and Shafi'i, are divided about when abortion is allowed. Jurists of the Hanafi School permit abortions until the 120th day. Jurists of the Hanbali School allow abortion up to the 40th day. Maliki School jurists also allow abortion up to the 40th day of pregnancy (but only with the consent of both parents of the woman), and the Shafi'i School allows abortions to be performed up to the 120th day.[5] However, Shia cleric Sistani says after implantation of the [fertilized] ovum [on the lining of the womb]...." abortion is never allowed.[6]

## Is Abortion Ever Sanctioned?

Most Islamic authorities agree that termination of pregnancy is defensible if the mother's life is in danger. In Islam, the life of the mother "with its responsibilities and ties takes precedence" over a fetus.[7] Qur'an 2:233 says, "…neither shall a mother be made to suffer because of her child …"

The Islamic legal maxim of the lesser of the two evils, also known as the more important and the less important, comes from a *hadith* of Prophet Muhammad: "When two forbidden things come [upon a person] together, then the lesser will be sacrificed for the greater."[8] Thus, saving the mother's life is more important than the life of the fetus. Sunni Shaykh Mahmud Shaltut says, "For the mother is the origin of the foetus [sic]; moreover, she is established in life, with duties and responsibilities, and she is also a pillar of the family. It would be not possible to sacrifice her life for the life of a feotus which has not yet acquired a personality and which has no responsibilities or obligations to fulfill."[9]

A number of jurists also permit abortion of physically or mentally defective fetuses before ensoulment. Some permit abortion only during the first three months of pregnancy, while others extend the "permission to abort a defective fetus to the first 120 days of pregnancy."[10] However, there are those who strongly argue against carte blanche abortion of fetuses with such physical challenges as blindness or the absence of a hand or a foot because they "may still lead a normal life."[11] Shia cleric Sistani prohibits abortions of deformed or defective fetuses and of fetuses expected to die soon after birth.[12]

Various jurists allow abortion of fetuses of mothers already nursing infants, who are unable to provide breast milk for both infants. In such a situation, the nursing infant has the right to life over the fetus. Before the development of infant feeding formulas, scholars stated that if the father of the child is able to pay for a wet nurse for the new child, abortion is not allowed. For most jurists, including Shia jurist Sistani, it is not acceptable for economic reasons to allow abortions.[13]

Moreover, most jurists do not permit women who are pregnant as a result of sexual assault to abort an unborn child. They do allow them to "use the morning after pill or RU486 immediately after the sexual assault to prevent pregnancy. If pregnant, however, they must carry the fetus to term. In such situations, Islam says, why abort the child for the crime of the father?"[14]

In closing, some Muslims point to Qur'an 6:151 as evidence that abortion is forbidden. It states, "…do not kill your children for fear of poverty? [for] it is We who shall provide sustenance for you as well as for them…" According to other scholars, this Qur'anic reference condemns only the ancient pre-Islamic custom of female infanticide.

## SUMMARY

### Sunni Schools of Islamic Law

The Sunni schools of Islamic law permit abortion should pregnancy threaten the mother's life or should a deformed or defective fetus be not viable enough to have a quality life. These abortions must be performed before the spirit (*ruh*) enters the fetus (ensoulment) up to day 40 or day 120, depending on the religious school of law.

• Hanafi School permits abortion until the 120th day.

• Hanbali School allows abortion up to the 40th day.

• Maliki School allows abortion up to the 40th day with the consent of both parents.

• Shafi'i School allows abortions to be performed up to the 120th day.

### Sunni Jurist Shaykh Yusuf Al-Qaradawi

• Abortion is *haram* "after the fetus is completely formed and has been given a soul."[15]

### Shia Jurist Ali Sistani

• Abortion is never allowed after the zygote is implanted on the lining of the womb.

• Deformed fetuses or those fetuses expected to die upon birth may not be aborted.

• Fetuses of economically destitute expectant women who are already nursing an infant may not be aborted.

### Islamic Medical Association of North America (IMANA)

• "Abortion may be permitted if continuation of pregnancy may cause the pregnant woman to die or cause serious deterioration of her health both medical and mental."

> The congenital conditions affecting [a] fetus in which abortions may be sought and may be permitted are lethal malformations

> not compatible with extra-uterine life .... But, even in these situations, it is preferable to do it before the [first] 120 days of pregnancy. In non-lethal situations, such as severe hydrocephaly, cervical spinal bifida, Down's syndrome, it may be permissible before 120 days of pregnancy after consulting Islamic scholars and medical experts in the field.[16]

• About victims of rape, war crimes, and incest, IMANA says, "In all cases, the recommendation [for abortion] should be made by a team of Islamic scholars and medical experts in the field."[17]

### Practical Steps for Caring for Muslim Patients

Some Islamic jurists allow abortions when pregnancy adversely affects the health of the woman or in cases of lethal fetal malformations. For voluntary termination of pregnancy (abortion), a patient and her family may need support in preparing for the death of the child. Remember, in Islam, after the ensoulment of a fetus, the fetus is a child. Conversely, before ensoulment, the fetus is not a child. If abortion takes place after ensoulment, follow the Islamic guidelines for burial; otherwise, there is no washing or funeral because the fetus is not human life. The same ensoulment rules and Islamic guidelines for burial preparation apply to involuntary abortion (miscarriage): before ensoulment, the fetus is not a child; but, after ensoulment, the fetus is a child. The following suggestions may be useful.

### Before Talking with the Patient and Family

1. Read the "Abortion" chapter.

2. Assess the patient's medical, emotional, and spiritual states. Check with those caring for the patient, including physicians, nurses, and chaplains.
3. Know the protocol of your hospital for the disposition of an aborted unensouled fetus. Alternatively, if a child dies after ensoulment, help the patient and family plan for the burial. See "Practical Steps at the Death of a Muslim Patient," Appendix 1.

### Once with the Patient and Family

1. Encourage the patient and her family to contact their religious leader for support or to seek the support of the healthcare chaplain.
2. Dealing with the termination of a pregnancy is often difficult. Some parents and their families may experience grief and/or guilt, among other feelings.
3. Speak alone with the patient and then with her family (husband, her husband's family and hers). Some families may want to be present during the initial patient consultation, but check with the patient first. You may ask the chaplain to find out about the patient's and family's faith beliefs and cultural mindsets regarding voluntary abortion. The family may have difficulty with the patient having an abortion, even though it is permitted and needed. Support the patient and her family.
4. The chaplain or healthcare worker should ask for permission to pray (*du'a*, sg./ *ad'iya*, pl.) for the needs of the patient and her family. Include Qur'anic verses (*ayat*) with the du'a. Find out which Qur'anic verse they prefer and if they want the chaplain or healthcare worker to read the scripture in English, or if they want to do the recitation themselves. Some Muslims are offended if a non-Muslim reads the Qur'an. See "Supplications (*ad'iya*)," Appendix 3.

5. Never ever invoke the name of Jesus in prayers; this is offensive to Muslims. Muslims pray only to God.
6. The chaplain or healthcare worker may suggest that the family repeat (*dhikr*) the names of God. See Appendix 8 for a list of God's names. *Dhikr* is a common spiritual practice among Muslims.
7. Assure the patient that God's mercy and love for both her and her fetus or child are unconditional, that she is acting according to her beliefs, and that generally in Islam the mother's life "with its responsibilities and ties, takes precedence" over a fetus.[18] Qur'an 2:233 says, "…neither shall a mother be made to suffer because of her child …"
8. Some Muslims may not want non-Muslims to touch a fetus or child. Check first with the parents or family spokesperson. Wearing surgical gloves may be a solution for healthcare providers needing to handle the remains.
9. Help the family to arrange to have an aborted fetus without a face or limbs, along with all tissue (placenta, etc.) wrapped in a cloth and buried. The family may want to shroud the fetus themselves. It should remain veiled. Allow for privacy during this ritual.
10. Islam does not allow cremation.
11. Many Muslims know that funeral prayer (*janazah*) is not required for an aborted fetus without a face and limbs. However, if the family wants *janazah* or to name the baby, there is no harm in doing so. Put the needs of the family first.
12. Help the family, if permitted by their sect's religious opinion, to arrange to have the aborted child with a face or limbs bathed (*ghusl*), shrouded (*kafan*), named, and buried after the funeral prayer (*janazah*).

The family may want to wash and shroud the child themselves. Allow for privacy during this ritual.

13. Most Muslims will want to say the name of Allah also known as the declaration of faith (*shahadah*) or the call to prayer (*adhan*) in the right ear of the child. This is not necessary. The child is in a state of purity. "Every child formed in a natural condition [*fitra*] in his mother's womb"[19] is in a state of purity, and is bound for Paradise (*janna*). The state of *fitra* is the "true and natural response to God, the innate religion of Islam."[20] However, if the parents want to say the name of Allah, or the declaration of faith (*shahadah*), or the call to prayer (*adhan*), there is no harm in doing so. Additionally, instead of saying these prayers in the right ear of the child, the parents could affirm their faith in God.

14. The *shahadah* is: "*ash-hadu an la ilaha illa Llah wa ash-hadu anna Muhammadan rasulu Llah*" or "I witness that there is no god but God, and I witness that Muhammad is the Messenger of God."

15. The *adhan* is: *allahu akbar* (said four times), *ash-hadu an la ilaha illa Llah* (said two times), *ash-hadu anna Muhammadan rasulu Llah* (said two times), *hayya 'ala al salat* (said two times), *hayya 'ala al falah* (said two times), *Allahu akbar* (said two times), *la ilaha illa Llah* (said one time): "God is greatest; I bear witness that there is no god but the One God; I bear witness that Muhammad is the Messenger of God; come fast to prayer; come fast to success; God is greatest; there is no god but the One God."

NOTES

[1] Yusuf Al-Qaradawi, *The Lawful and the Prohibited in Islam,* trans. Kamal El-Helbawy, M. Moinuddin Siddiqui, Syed Shukry (Indianapolis, IN: American Trust Publications, 1982), 201 (hereinafter cited as Qaradawi, *The Lawful*).

[2] Hereafter the Shia cleric's name is transliterated as "Sistani."

[3] Muhammad ibn Ismail al-Bukhari, *Sahih Bukhari* 4:549. See also, *Sahih al-Boukhari, Being the Traditions of Sayings and Doings of the Prophet Muhammad As Narrated By His Companions,* Vol. IX, rendered to English by Mahmoud Matraji, corrected and revised by F. Amira Zrein Matraji (Beirut, Lebanon: Dar El Aker, 1993), 16-17/35-37.

[4] Vardit Rispler-Chaim, *Islamic Medical Ethics in the Twentieth Century* (Leiden: E.J. Brill, 1993), 9.

[5] Kiarash Aramesh, "Abortion: An Islamic Ethical View," *Iranian Journal of Allergy, Asthma and Immunology* 6, Suppl. 5 (February 2007):31.

[6] Rispler-Chaim, 15.

[7] A.R. Gatrad and A. Sheikh, "Medical ethics and Islam: principles and practice," *Archives of Disease in Childhood* 84 (2001): 74.

[8] Sayyid Muhammad Rizvi, *Marriage and Morals in Islam* (Scarborough, Ontario, Canada: Islamic Education and Information Center, 1990), 111.

[9] Qaradawi, *The Lawful,* 202.

[10] Rispler-Chaim, 14-15.

[11] Ibid., 15.

[12] Ayatullah Ali al-Husaini as-Seestani, *A Code of Practice for Muslims in the West,* trans. Sayyid Muhammad Rizvi (London, England: Imam Ali Foundation, 1999), 222 (#447). (Note: Some publishers transliterate the Shia cleric's name as Seestani; however, this paper uses the transliteration of "Sistani.")

[13] Sistani, 221-22 (446-48).

[14] Rizvi, 111.

[15] Qaradawi, *The Lawful,* 89.

[16] IMANA Ethics Committee, "Islamic Medical Ethics," available at the website of the Islamic Society of North America, http://www.isna.net/Leadership/pages/Islamic-Medical-Ethics.aspx. Accessed 19 February 2010.

[17] Ibid.

[18] Gatrad and Sheikh, "Medical ethics": 74.

[19] Jane I. Smith and Yvonne Yazbeck Haddad, *The Islamic Understanding of Death and Resurrection* (New York: Oxford University Press, 2002), 172.

[20] Ibid. Note: In Islam, children become accountable for their own faith and actions at the age of puberty.

# CHAPTER 8

# AUTOPSY

Abdullah, age 16, drowns while swimming alone in a river near his home. An ambulance takes his body to the county medical examiner's office, and the police notify his parents, Aisha and Yahya. They also are told that state law requires autopsy in cases of accidental deaths. However, in accordance with their Muslim faith, Aisha and Yahya ask that the procedure not be performed, and ultimately, seek an injunction (though without success) to prevent it.

Muslims generally refuse autopsy for deceased family members because they believe that everything – including death – is God's will; therefore, knowledge about the cause of death is theologically useless. Moreover, most believe that autopsy desecrates the dead, and some believe the dead experience physical pain. Also, Muslims generally bury their deceased loved ones as soon as possible after death.[1]

## Islamic Perspective on Autopsy

The issue of autopsy is not addressed specifically in the two primary sources of Islamic law or *shari'a*, which is based on the Qur'an and the authenticated actions and words (*Sunna*) of Prophet Muhammad. Autopsy did not exist during the lifetime of Prophet Muhammad. However, Islamic jurists' legal opinions (*fatwas*) on autopsy reflect the underlying principles of the Qur'an and *Sunna*. The *fatwas* in this book are from two leading jurists, Ali Sistani, a Shiite, and Shaykh Yusuf Qaradawi, a Sunni. They both state that autopsy should be avoided, if possible. As noted in the earlier anecdote about the drowned boy, Muslims believe that God ordains the time of death; some believe that the dead experience physical pain and that autopsy desecrates the body of the deceased. "The position of all Shiite jurists, including [Ali] Sistani … is that an autopsy is considered to be a desecration of the body; it is a practice that is abhorred and to be refused by the family if requested."[2]

Autopsy can delay burial. Prophet Muhammad counseled "not waiting for morning to bury if the person died at night; and not waiting for nightfall if the person died in the morning. Make haste in taking them to their resting place."[3]

Despite the forgoing principles opposing autopsy, there are two primary exceptions. According to Shia jurist Sistani and Sunni jurists Qaradawi, autopsies may be performed if required by law or if beneficial to medical science for the purpose of saving lives.[4]

In the first case, should state law require autopsy to determine the cause of death, the family of the deceased must comply. Because they have no choice in the matter, say the jurists, they are not accountable for the body's disfigurement on the Day of Judgment.[5]

In the second instance, autopsy may be permitted if knowledge gathered from it leads to new lifesaving medical technologies and treatments. (This should be communicated to the family of the deceased as soon as possible). The *fatwa* of Shia jurist Sistani states: "It is not permissible to perform autopsy on the body of a dead Muslim for the sake of education and other purposes. It is only permissible, if the life of another Muslim depends on it – even if it is sometime in the future." [6]

Years before Sistani's *fatwa*, the supreme head of the Islamic School of Jurisprudence in Egypt in 1952 issued a precedent-setting *fatwa*. It states that "if anything was of 'good' for humanity then 'necessity allows what is prohibited.'" Thirty years later, another *fatwa* committee "found that the benefits of autopsies outweighed the drawbacks if they increase the knowledge of medical students and doctors, help control contagious diseases, and serve the cause of justice." [7]

## PRIMARY ISSUES AND BELIEFS ABOUT AUTOPSY

### Can Autopsy Advance Medical Science?

In the following celebrated saying, Prophet Muhammad encouraged Muslims to learn and apply their knowledge for the benefit of all: "The seeking of knowledge is obligatory for every Muslim." [8] Islam also emphasizes and encourages scientific investigation. Qur'an 51:20-21 says, "On the earth are signs [of God's existence, visible] for those of assured Faith, as also in your own selves: Will ye not then see?"

Despite ample evidence proving that information gathered from autopsies fulfills these requirements and contributes to patient services, research, and public health, the number of autopsies performed on Muslims worldwide has been declining for decades[9] for many of the reasons already mentioned. In addition, in Islam, scientific knowledge does not take precedence over religious obligations and the dignity of the human being. Because Muslims understand the value of scientific knowledge differently, and place great weight on their obligation to protect the deceased from indignity, usually they are reluctant to permit autopsies.

### Does Autopsy Desecrate the Body of the Deceased?

In Qur'an 17:70, God says, "Now indeed, We have conferred dignity on the children of Adam, and borne them over land and sea, and provided for them sustenance out of the good things of life, and favoured them far above most of Our creation."

As emphasized in the *ayah*, the dignity of human beings is of the utmost importance. In Islam, this extends to the dead. The body of the deceased is a person, not just a corpse. As such, the body should not be desecrated by embalming, cosmetic touch-ups, or other funerary procedures and trappings.

Yet, Islam also ascribes great significance to the purpose or intention (*niyya*) of every action. One of the five core maxims of Islam[10] at the very center of the hundreds of other maxims in Islamic law is matters will be judged by their purposes. "Actions and activities are not done for their sake alone; it is not enough to 'go through the motions...'" As mentioned above, the maxim's wording is based on the *hadith*: "Acts are judged only by intentions."[11] Therefore, postmortem examination is not desecration if the purpose is to benefit medical science and subsequently humankind or to comply with the law of the land; additionally, autopsy is not desecration if families find comfort in knowing what caused the death of their love one.

### Do the Deceased Feel Pain?

The answer to this question depends on interpretation. The Qur'an does not say whether the dead experience physical pain; however, a *hadith* states: "Breaking the bones of the deceased is like breaking it when he was alive."[12] Some Muslims take this literally, while others say the "text obliges the Muslim community to deal humanely with fellow human beings whether in life or in death." [13]

### Can Burial Be Delayed Because of Autopsy?

Muslims' belief in the dignity of the dead reflects their practice of prompt burial. Muslims bury the body usually within 24 hours of death because Prophet Muhammad counseled, "not waiting for morning to bury if the person died at night; and not waiting for nightfall if the person died in the morning. Make haste in taking them to their resting place."[14] This respectfully enables the body to begin decomposition in the earth. Should a postmortem examination be required, however, it should be performed within 24 hours of death, or as soon as feasibly possible. Muslims consider embalming, cosmetic touch-ups or other funerary trappings forms of mutilation and disrespectful of the bodies of their deceased loved ones.

### Summary

1. Islam's prohibition against autopsy is based on the following beliefs: the body should not be cut into or desecrated.
2. Some Muslims also believe the dead feel pain.
3. Burial should take place within 24 hours whenever possible: by evening, if the person dies in the morning and by morning, if he or she dies at night. A speedy burial usually does not allow time for an autopsy.
4. Leading Muslim jurists have ruled that autopsy is permissible when required by law. In such cases, the family has no choice; therefore, they are not held accountable by Islamic law.
5. Autopsy is permissible if it leads to knowledge that could benefit medical science and help save lives now and in the future.
6. How a person or community interprets the prohibitions influences beliefs about autopsy.
7. Autopsies can take up to several days. The person conducting the autopsy should be told about the family's faith needs.
8. After the autopsy, removed body parts should be reattached to their original locations, and if this is not possible, should be placed within the body. The body should be wrapped in clean sheets and returned to the family for burial.
9. Muslims do not want the bodies of loved ones embalmed or tampered with in any other way.
10. Do not cut the nails and hair of the deceased person.

## PRACTICAL STEPS FOR CARING FOR MUSLIM PATIENTS

The body of the deceased must be treated respectfully. In Islam, opinions about autopsy are complex and vary culturally, religiously, and personally. The primary focus of the chaplain or healthcare worker should be those grieving the loss of a loved one.

### Before Talking with the Family of the Deceased

1. Read the "Autopsy" chapter.
2. Become familiar with the circumstances surrounding the patient's death. Did the patient die accidentally, from illness, or from other causes? Ask the involved healthcare providers for an assessment of the situation and the family's emotional and spiritual states.
3. Find out about the local and state autopsy laws.
4. Become familiar with the hospital's procedures for the release of a dead body.
5. Have funeral- and burial-planning information available for the family. See "Practical Steps at Death of a Muslim Patient," Appendix 1.

### Once with the Family of the Deceased

1. Encourage the family to contact their imam or religious leader for support.
2. Ask about the family's cultural and religious beliefs with regard to autopsy.
3. Determine and provide support specific to the family's physical, emotional, and spiritual needs.
4. Make sure the family knows that their need for quick burial and proper handling of their loved one is understood and has been heard by healthcare workers.

5. Be aware that anxiety about autopsy may stem from personal interpretations, not from Islam.
6. Explain that if the law requires autopsy, they must comply; therefore, they are not accountable for what happens to the body as the result of autopsy, according to the *shari'a*. Tell them that those conducting the autopsy will do so with the greatest respect for their loved one.
7. Help them understand that in Islam, performing an autopsy to advance medical science in order to save the lives of others or to improve the health of others is highly beneficial.
8. Explain that autopsy could uncover the cause of the death of their loved one, which could be comforting to them.
9. If the family is concerned about their deceased loved one feeling the pain of autopsy, explain that according to most Islamic jurists, the dead do not feel physical pain. Otherwise, the decaying process also would be painful.
10. Chaplains or non-family members or friends should ask for permission to pray (*du'a*) for the needs of the deceased. Include Qur'anic verses (*ayat*) with the *du'a*. See "Supplications (*ad'iya*)," Appendix 3. Find out which *ayah* they prefer, if they want someone to read the verses in English or if they prefer to recite them. Some Muslims are offended if a non-Muslim reads the Qur'an. Never invoke the name of Jesus; this is offensive to Muslims, who pray only to God.
11. Some Muslims may want to repeat (*dhikr*) the names of God. See Appendix 8 for a list of God's names.
12. Other Muslims recite Qur'an 36 (*Ya-Sin*) for their deceased loved one at the bedside and at the burial. Make sure this is culturally acceptable to the family. Provide the *sura*, or help the family get a CD of the sura. See Qur'an 36 (*Ya-Sin*) Appendix 3.

NOTES

[1] Mudher al-Adnani and Irene Scheimberg, "How can we improve the rate of autopsies among Muslims?" *British Medical Journal* 332 (4 February 2006): 310.

[2] Jonathan E. Brockopp and Thomas Eich, eds., *Muslim Medical Ethics: From Theory to Practice* (Columbia, S.C.: University of South Carolina Press, 2008), 174.

[3] Abdul Sachedina, *Islamic Biomedical Ethics: Principles and Applications* (Oxford: Oxford University Press, 2009), 176 (hereinafter cited as "Abdul Sachedina").

[4] Brockopp and Eich, ibid.

[5] Ibid.

[6] Ali Sistani, *A Code of Practice for Muslims in the West,* trans. Sayyid Muhammad Rizvi (London, England: Imam Ali Foundation, 1999), 189 (347).

[7] Al-Adnani and Scheimberg, 310.

[8] Al-Tirmidhi, *hadith* 74, in K.S. Durrany, *Impact of Islamic fundamentalism* (Delhi: Christian Institute for the Study of Religion and Society, 1993), 77.

[9] Olayiwola Abideen Oluwasola, FWACP; Olufunmilayo I. Fawole, FMCPH; Abiodun Jesse Otegbayo, FWACP; Gabriel Olabiyi Ogun, FNCP; Clement A. Adebamowo, DSc; Afolabi Elijah Bamigboye, Ph.D., "The Autopsy: Knowledge, Attitude, and Perceptions of Doctors and Relatives of the Deceased," *Pathology and Laboratory Medicine* 133, No. 1 (January 2009): 78–82.

[10] Five core maxims: Matters will be judged by their purposes, certainty will not be overturned by doubt, harm must be removed, hardship must be alleviated, and custom has the weight of law. Umar Faruq Abd-Allah, "Living Islam with Purpose" (Nawawi Foundation Paper, 2007), 23, http://www.nawawi.org/downloads/article6.pdf. Accessed 20 November 2009.

[11] Ibid.

[12] Narrated by Abu Dawood (2792), in Abu Da'ud Sulayman ibn al-Ash'ath al-Sijistani, *Sunan Abu Dawud,* Vol. 4 (Beirut, Lebanon: Dar al-Kotob al-Ilmiyah Publishing House, 2008), 26.

[13] A.R. Gatrad and A. Sheikh, "Medical ethics and Islam: principles and practice," *Archives of Disease in Childhood* 84 (2001):72-75. See also Muhammad ibn Ismail al-Bukhari, *Sahih Bukhari,* Vol. 8, 175 ("Do not abuse the dead, for they have reached the result of what they have done."), University of Southern California *ahadith* database:
http://www.usc.edu/schools/college/crcc/engagement/resources/texts/muslim/hadith/bukhari/052.sbt.html. Accessed 4 April 2010.

[14] Abdul Sachedina, 176.

# CHAPTER 9

# CIRCUMCISION

A 6-year old girl's Turkish mother refuses to have her daughter circumcised; however, the girl's father, who comes from a village in rural Africa, thinks differently. He wants to continue his village's tradition of circumcising females during their seventh year, but as a recent immigrant to the U.S., he is eager to adopt the ways of his new country and he also wants to please his wife. He consults with a female Muslim pediatrician. He learns that circumcision is not a simple, harmless procedure for females, but that part, or all, of the sexual organ is removed, which can cause long-term serious health problems. He also finds out that in California, where he and his family live, female circumcision is against the law.

The practice of female circumcision, according to anecdotal evidence from medical practitioners in the U.S. (factual information is unavailable), is uncommon among America-born Muslims, but is common among grown immigrant women circumcised in their countries of origin. The vast majority of Muslims worldwide do not believe in female circumcision. Most countries have outlawed female circumcision.

## Islamic Perspective on Circumcision

Some practitioners of female genital cutting, euphemistically called circumcision (*khafd*), look for supporting evidence in the *hadith* literature, because the subject matter does not appear in the Qur'an. A popular *hadith* states:

"circumcision is *Sunna* (obligatory) for men and charity (good deeds) for women, but various sources do not consider that *hadith* as authentic."[1] There is an authentic *hadith*, however, that says Prophet Muhammad instructed a woman who performed circumcision in Medina not to "cut severely as that is better for a woman and more desirable for a husband."[2] Some scholars, nevertheless, determined that this *hadith* addresses pre-Islamic tribes during the early years of Islam. These tribes had been practicing circumcision long before the arrival of Islam.[3] The converts to Islam had carried this ritual, among others, into their new faith tradition. It is a tenet of Islam not to impose itself on the customs of people, but rather to gently guide them to a better way.

The legal opinions (*fatwas*) of the four major Sunni schools of jurisprudence are as follows: Maliki School jurists "allegedly" do not consider female circumcision "a sin if it is not performed."[4] Hanbali School jurists "allegedly" say female circumcision is "sunna (good practice, as exemplified by the Prophet), that is, less than obligatory but very strongly encouraged."[5] Shafi'i School jurists "allegedly" consider female circumcision obligatory.[6] However, renowned Mahmud Shaltut of the Hanafi School finds "no legal justification of any kind to perform female circumcision."[7] He refutes all arguments, medical, ethical, and from *Shari'a* that support circumcision. Thus, it cannot be justified as a "protective measure against sexual temptations for women,"[8] nor can it, or any other physical measure, guarantee chastity.[9] Additionally, Mohamed Magid, executive director of the All Dulles Area Muslim Society (ADAMS) in Washington, D.C., and president of the Islamic Society of North America, says, "Islam discourages female circumcision because the harm is more than the benefit. Medically, it has been proven that the procedure causes complications that hurt the patient, emotionally and physically. Many Muslim healthcare providers in Muslim countries have recommended this not be practiced at all."[10]

In the U.S., immigrant non-Muslim and Muslim parents circumcise about 2,000 of their daughters every year, and most of these surgeries, often without anesthesia, take place in unsterilized environments. Worldwide, more than 150 million infants to adults in more than 30 countries in Africa, Asia, and the Middle East have suffered the painful and highly dangerous practice of the removal of all or part of the external female genitalia.[11] Health hazards of female circumcision include:

1. Immediate (including pain, hemorrhage, shock, acute urinary retention, urinary infection, blood poisoning, fever, tetanus, death and fracture of clavicle); delayed healing, pelvic infection, cysts and abscesses, keloid scar, painful intercourse
2. Late complications (including closure of the vaginal opening by the scar tissue, infertility, recurrent urinary tract infection, difficulty in urinating, stone formation, hypersensitivity, and incontinence and fissure)
3. In consummation (difficulty in penetration, fear of the sex act, failure of the circumcision scar to dilate)
4. At delivery (prolonged and obstructed labor, unnecessary Caesarian section, other gynecological consequences, stillbirth, emotionally handicapped children, etc.)
5. Postnatal complications (miscarriages, descent of uterus into the vagina)
6. Sexual problems (lack of orgasm, frigidity, anxiety, depression, temporary impotence and frustration over long-lasting inability to consummate marriage)[12]

On the other hand, most Muslim boys undergo circumcision before puberty at an age set by parents and religious leaders. Some Shiite jurists determine the age to be seven days, which is when they say Prophet Muhammad circumcised his two grandsons, Hassan and Husayn.[13] Others prefer deferring the procedure to about 10, the age of legal responsibility, saying that no boy should have to suffer pain until he reaches that age.[14] Most Muslim parents have their male infants circumcised shortly after birth in the hospital. There are no established religious ceremonies or prayers pertaining to circumcision; however, there are many diverse cultural practices and celebrations associated with circumcision.

There is consensus among Islamic scholars that circumcision (*khitan*) is required of Muslim males. Additionally, a number of authentic (*sahih*) reports of the words and actions of Prophet Muhammad (*ahadith*) mention *khitan*. One *hadith* has to do with Prophet Abraham, who in obedience to a command from God, at age 80, used an adze to circumcise himself (*khitan*).[15/16] The Qur'an does not mention the circumcision of males.

According to Islamic tradition, Prophet Abraham was the first circumcised Muslim.[17] Another *hadith* includes circumcision, which historically has been thought to provide a modicum of protection against infections, among other hygienic practices established by Prophet Muhammad. A companion of Prophet Muhammad, Abu Huraira, narrated, "I heard the Prophet saying. 'Five practices are characteristics of the *fitra* [natural way]: circumcision, shaving the pubic hair, cutting the moustaches short, clipping the nails, and depilating the hair of the armpits.'"[18]

The legitimacy of the practice of male circumcision from Prophet Muhammad greatly influences the legal rulings (*fatwas*) of Islamic jurists. The *fatwas* of jurists of the four Sunni schools of jurisprudence are as follows: Male circumcision is an obligation (*fard*) with the Shafi'i School; the Hanafi School recommends male circumcision; the Maliki and Hanbali schools permit the practice. Most Shiite jurists say male circumcision is obligatory. Exemptions apply to sickly baby boys, those born circumcised, and elderly and infirm male converts.[19]

## SUMMARY

### Female Circumcision

1. Genital cutting, also known as female genital mutilation or circumcision (*khafd*), involves the removal of all or part of the external female genitalia.
2. Maliki School jurists "allegedly" do not consider female circumcision "a sin if it is not performed."[20] Hanbali School jurists "allegedly" say it is "*sunna* (good practice, as exemplified by the Prophet), that is, less than obligatory but very strongly encouraged."[21] Shafi'i School jurists "allegedly" consider it obligatory. No English translation was available with regard to the Hanafi School's position on female circumcision.
3. Sunni cleric Mahmud Shaltut ruled that there is no Islamic legal justification for female circumcision.
4. Parents determine the age at which to circumcise their child.
5. There are no Islamic ceremonies or prayers associated with the practice of circumcision.

### Male Circumcision

1. Male circumcision involves removing the foreskin of the penis.
2. Male circumcision is considered obligatory by the Shafi'i School of jurisprudence, is recommended by the Hanafi School of jurisprudence, and is permitted by the Maliki and Hanbali schools of jurisprudence.
3. Exempt from circumcision are sickly baby boys, those born circumcised, and elderly and infirm male converts.
4. The age of circumcision varies from birth to 10.
5. There are no Islamic ceremonies or prayers associated with the practice of circumcision.

### Practical Steps for Caring for Muslim Patients

Many states outlaw female circumcision; however, this does not prevent well-intentioned parents from having the procedure performed by someone in their community. Male circumcision, on the other hand, is a regular practice among most Muslims and does not have deleterious effects.

### Before Talking with the Girl's Parents

1. Read the "Circumcision" chapter.
2. Become familiar with state laws on female circumcision.

### Once with the Girl's Parents

1. Encourage the family to contact their imam or religious leader for support.
2. Check the family's faith beliefs and cultural sensitivities concerning female circumcision.
3. Explain that female circumcision is not a simple, harmless procedure. If

needed, ask a physician to explain the health and emotional risks of female circumcision.

4. Point out that Islam does not condone female circumcision, that there is no proof in the Qur'an or *Sunna* (actions and words of Prophet Muhammad) that supports this practice, that Islamic scholars do not recommend it, that female circumcision existed long before the advent of Islam, and that this cultural practice entwined with Islam centuries ago and has survived to modern times.

5. Generally, sexual-related issues should be discussed with the parents, not with the child or teen. Be discerning. Put the safety and well-being of the underage patient first.

### Before Talking with the Boy's Parents

1. Read the "Circumcision" chapter.

### Once with the Boy's Parents

1. Encourage family to contact their imam or religious leader for support.
2. Find out about the family's beliefs and cultural sensitivities about male circumcision.
3. If warranted, ask a physician to explain that scientific evidence shows inconclusive medical benefits from male circumcision.
4. Support the parent's decision to have their son circumcised by referring to the practice (*Sunna*) of Prophet Muhammad. Mention that Prophet Abraham was the first to perform this rite.
5. Explain that this procedure, according to *Sunna*, is usually performed seven days after the birth of the child. This is part of the welcoming consecration

(*aqiqah*) ritual. See "Welcoming a newborn baby (*aqiqah*)," Appendix 2. However, advocate on behalf of the parents to have this procedure performed on the seventh day or any other date of their choosing, should the physician or other healthcare providers suggest that circumcision be done upon birth or before the seventh day.

6. Advocate on behalf of a sickly or premature newborn boy to delay circumcision. Explain that while circumcision on the seventh day is recommended, it is not obligatory. In Islam, the well-being of the child is greater than the act of circumcision, and this practice can be completed when the child is healthy.[22]

---

NOTES

[1] Hassan Hathout, "Female Circumcision Is NOT Required by Islam," at Islamic Research Foundation International, http://www.irfi.org/articles/articles_1751_1800/female%20circumcision%20is%20not%20required%20by%20islamhtml.htm. Accessed 8 December 2009.

[2] Abu Dawud, *Sunan Abu Dawud,* Book 41, No. 5251, from the University of Southern California's *ahadith* database: http://www.usc.edu/schools/college/crcc/engagement/resources/texts/muslim/hadith/abudawud/041.sat.html. Accessed 8 December 2009.

[3] Sangeeta Dhami and Aziz Sheikh, "The family: predicament and promise," in *Caring for Muslim Patients*, 2nd ed. Eds. Aziz Sheikh and Abdul Rashid Gatrad (Oxon, United Kingdom: Radcliffe Publishing, 2009), 63.

[4] Vardit Rispler-Chaim, *Islamic Medical Ethics in the Twentieth Century* (Leiden: E.J. Brill, 1993), 86.

[5] Ibid.

[6] Ibid. Research was unable to locate English translations of the *fatwa* of the Shia jurist Ali Sistani concerning female circumcision.

[7] Rispler-Chaim, 86.

[8] Ibid, 90.

[9] Ibid.

[10] Phone interview with Mohamed Magid, executive director of the All Dulles Area Muslim Society (ADAMS) in Washington, D.C., and president of the Islamic Society of North America, February 10, 2010.

[11] International Federation of Gynecology and Obstetrics (IFGO), "Warning issued over 'unnecessary' vaginal surgery," http://www.figo.org/projects/general_assembly_resolution_FGM. Accessed 9 December 2009. Note: The IFGO passed a resolution calling for the ban of female circumcision. Visit http://www.figo.org/projects/general_assembly_resolution_FGM to view the resolution.

[12] Rispler-Chaim, 91.

[13] Ibid., 87.

[14] Ibid.

[15] Muhammad ibn Ismail al-Bukhari, *Sahih Bukhari,* Volume 4, Book 55, Number 575, University of Southern California *ahadith* database: http://www.usc.edu/schools/college/crcc/engagement/resources/texts/muslim/hadith/bukhari/055.sbt.html. Accessed 7 December 2009. "Narrated Abu Huraira: Allah's Apostle said, 'Abraham did his circumcision with an adze at the age of eighty.'"

[16] Massoume Price, "Rituals of Circumcision," December 2001, at the website of Culture of Iran,

http://74.125.93.132/search?q=cache:MQpXgeso55sJ:www.iranchamber.com/culture/articles/rituals_of_circumcision.php+%22Oceans+of+Light%22+and+circumcision&cd=1&hl=en&ct=clnk&gl=usL. Accessed 9 December 2009. From that site, the following text comes: "A *hadith* attributed to 'Ali reports, Abraham was told: Cleanse/Purify yourself, so he trimmed his moustache. Then he was told: Cleanse/purify yourself, and he plucked the hair from under his arms. Then he was told: Cleanse/Purify yourself, and he shaved his pubic area, then he was told: Cleanse/Purify yourself, and he circumcised himself." (Bihar al-Anwar). Other *ahadith* say that Prophet Adam was the first circumcised person.

[17] Complete *Malik's Muwatta,* Book 49, Number 49.3.4: "Yahya related to me from Malik from Yahya ibn Said that Said ibn al-Musayyub said, 'Ibrahim, may Allah bless him and grant him peace, was the first to give hospitality to the guest and the first person to be circumcised and the first person to trim the moustache and the first person to see grey hair. He said, 'O Lord! What is this?' Allah the Blessed, the Exalted, said, 'It is dignity, Ibrahim.' He said, 'Lord, increase me in dignity!''" This *hadith* is from the University of Southern California *ahadith* database: http://www.usc.edu/schools/college/crcc/engagement/resources/texts/muslim/hadith/muwatta/049.mmt.html. Accessed 7 December 2009.

[18] Muhammad ibn Ismail al-Bukhari, *Sahih Bukhari,* Volume 7, Book 72, Number 779, University of Southern California *ahadith* database: http://www.usc.edu/schools/college/crcc/engagement/resources/texts/muslim/hadith/bukhari/072.sbt.html. Accessed 7 December 2009.

[19] Rispler-Chaim, 88.

[20] Ibid.

[21] Ibid.

[22] Imam Magid interview, Feb. 10, 2010.

# CHAPTER 10

# DEATH AND DYING

After three years of radiation, chemotherapy, and surgeries, Amma is dying. Her battle with cancer is about to end. The oncologist has confirmed that she has days, if not hours, remaining. Despite the prescribed medications, Amma is in excruciating pain and alert. Friends had been calling and visiting, but now only her devoted and caring husband, Aziz, their three grown children, and two of her most devout friends are at her bedside. They are there to help her transition from this life to the next by gently encouraging her to seek forgiveness for any wrongdoings, recall her good deeds, and remember that God is the All-Merciful and All-Compassionate.

Amma has reacted as would be expected of anyone in her situation: with grief, regret, and, on more than one occasion, fear, anger, and hopelessness. She has done the emotional and spiritual work privately with family, close friends, a counselor, and prayerfully with her Lord. The fruits of that work – a state of patience, calm, and equanimity of spirit – are evident. Even now, as she dies a painful death, Amma remains in this equanimous state, which could be interpreted by others as a flat affect or one of long-suffering. However, these assumptions would be incorrect. The truth is that Amma believes that this life is not her final abode and that now is her appointed time to die. It is the will of God. These beliefs comfort her.

## Islamic Perspective on Death and Dying

Islam is a way of life for Muslims, and it is a way of dying. The following are core elements of this way of being.

## Time of Death Is Set by and Known Only to God

Muslims understand that, as part of the overall divine plan, there is an appointed time (*ajal*) of death for everyone and that when their time is up, they have to go. Because of this belief, Muslims do not fight with fate. At the same time, they also believe in the sanctity of life, which is why they do everything possible to get well or to recover from injury. Medicine is a tool or means of healing, but the actual healing, Muslims believe, comes from God.

> Now [as for me, I know that,] verily, these [false deities] are my enemies, [and that none is my helper] save the Sustainer of all the worlds, who has created me and is the One who guides me, and is the One who gives me to eat and to drink, and when I fall ill, is the One who restores me to health and who will cause me to die and then will bring me back to life. (Qur'an 77-80)

Nevertheless, when death approaches Muslims embrace the finality of their physical existence with a sense of acceptance. In Qur'an 3:145, God says, "And no human being can die save by God's leave, at a term pre-ordained." And, Qur'an 39:42 states:

> It is God [alone that has this power – He] who causes all human beings to die at the time of their [bodily] death, and [causes to be as dead], during their sleep, those that have not yet died: thus, He withholds [from life] those upon whom He has decreed death, and lets

> the others go free for a term set [by Him]. In [all] this, behold, there are messages indeed for people who think!

Coexisting with the concept of fate is free will. Muslims believe that their choices are theirs alone, as are the consequences. That is, they are responsible for what they do, and will be held accountable for their choices on the Day of Resurrection.

> Every human being is bound to taste death: but only on the Day of Resurrection will you be requited in full [for whatever you have done] – whereupon [one] that shall be drawn away from the fire and brought into paradise will indeed have gained a triumph: for the life of this world is nothing but the enjoyment of self-delusion. (Qur'an 3:185)

A particularly poignant report (*hadith*) states that Prophet Muhammad said, "Verily, the first thing Allah created was the Pen, right after that He commanded it 'Record!' and the Pen recorded everything that will occur until the Day of Resurrection." (Al-Timidhi and Abu Dawud).[1]

## Death Marks the Beginning of Eternal Life

Belief in the Afterlife (*akhira*) is another central doctrine of Islam, and the Qur'an and *Sunna* (actions and words of Prophet Muhammad) describe the various conditions of the deceased in Paradise (*janna*) and Hell. From these holy texts, Muslims discern that death releases them from life's burdens. For Muslims, death is when the soul (*ruh*) departs the body. Muslims believe that they have only one physical life, but they exist forever as spiritual beings. Death then is an entryway to eternal life: "And [as for all such believers,] no human being can imagine what blissful delights, as yet hidden, await them [in the life to come] as a reward for all that they did." (Qur'an 32:17) For Muslims, death marks the transition from one existence to another. The transition from impermanent existence to eternal life finds expression in various languages, such as Urdu, a language of Pakistan and India. The word for death in Urdu is *intecal*, which means to transfer from this realm to the other.[2] The connection, therefore, is clear for Muslims – death is inevitable and so is the Afterlife; both can be a source of hope.

### Life and Death Have Purpose

All of life is a cosmic challenge to Muslims. They are ever mindful that life on earth is serious business and it is brief – because what they do here weighs heavily on their spiritual placement in the Hereafter (Paradise for pious Muslims and Hell for sinners). "Islam teaches that life on earth is an examination–the life to come is the eternal abode where one will reap the fruit of one's endeavors on earth..."[3]

Prophet Muhammad said, "The world is a sowing field for the other world. Therefore, sow this seed for now is the time to sow. You have land and water, so scatter seeds abroad. Act like a farmer and be busy with this work. If you don't till the grainfield, then you won't be worth half a millet seed on that threshing floor."[4] Therefore, for the sake of spiritual maturity, Islamic teachings encourage Muslims to strive for righteousness in the face of hardship. Guidelines for living a pious life are found in the Qur'an and the exemplary life of Prophet Muhammad (*Sunna*). Muslims reference these sources for shaping their own personal and social codes of conduct.

As with living, dying is also a test of the resolve of Muslims to be in alignment with their faith. Dying offers many opportunities for right conduct and profound meaning. This includes an accounting of deeds, drawing to a close of special relationships, and seeking of reconciliation and forgiveness from and of others, themselves and God. "Al-Nawawi, the famous traditionalist, is reported to have said that a dying person must hope for God's forgiveness and mercy and know that God is not keen to punish him: he should recite the Qur'anic verses and Hadiths from the Prophet that speak of hope and divine mercy." [5]

Dying, then, is considered a trial (*bala*) of this worldly life in preparation for eternal life: "Hallowed be He in whose hand all dominion rests, since He has the power to will anything: He who has created death as well as life, so that He might put you to a test [and thus show] which of you is best in conduct, and [make you realize that] He alone is almighty, truly forgiving." (Qur'an 67: 1-2) The hardship of dying also can be a catalyst for drawing a person spiritually closer to God in order that they may experience the divine mercy and compassion, as can be seen by the following report (*hadith*): "When Prophet Muhammad was dying, he put his hands in a large cup of water that was close to him and wiped his face with it, saying: 'O Allah help me over the hardship and agony of death.'" (Al-Tirmidhi). [6]

## Summary

The time of death is set by and known only to God. The death of the body is not the end of life. It marks the beginning of eternal life. Life and death have purpose.

## Practical Steps for Caring for Muslim Patients

Muslims believe that death is the next stage before the Day of Judgment. In the hospital room, the dying person prepares for this transition. The patient faces toward *Al-Ka'ba*, the first and most ancient house of worship in Islam, which is in Mecca, Saudi Arabia. It is toward *Al-Ka'ba* that Muslims direct their five daily ritual prayers (*salah*). Many family members and friends gather around the patient to encourage their loved one to draw closer to God. Dying is a time of great dignity and respect and holiness for Muslims. It is a family affair.

## Before Talking with the Family of the Dying or Deceased

1. Gather information from the physician and nurses about the dying or deceased patient's medical, emotional, and spiritual states.
2. Understand the hospital guidelines for releasing the body.
3. Become familiar with the "Islamic Perspective on Death and Dying" section.
4. Have available funeral information for the family. See "Practical Steps at Death of a Muslim Patient," Appendix 1.

## Once at the Bedside of the Dying or Deceased and with the Family

1. Encourage the family to contact their imam or religious leader for support.
2. Arrange to have the dying patient moved to face toward *Al-Ka'ba* in Mecca, Saudi Arabia, the house of worship reported to have been built by prophets Abraham and Ishmael and the direction of prayer (*salah*) for Muslims worldwide.

3. Remind the patient and the patient's family that God ("Allah" is the Arabic name for God) is the All-Merciful, All-Compassionate, and All-Forgiving.
4. Assure the family that in Islam, life eternal is just beyond this temporal dispensation. Share with them, but not in front of their loved one, that now may be their loved one's appointed time to die. In some cultures, it is not appropriate to talk about death in front of a dying person. Emphasis should be on helping the dying person to focus on God.
5. Chaplains or others, as they feel comfortable, may want to soothe the dying person by making supplication (*du'a*) to God. Ask the patient and/or the patient's family which supplication they prefer. Find out if they would like to recite the *du'a* in Arabic or if they prefer you to read it in English.
6. Be aware that some Muslims are offended if a non-Muslim reads the Qur'an.
7. Never ever invoke the name of Jesus in prayers; this is offensive to Muslims. Muslims pray only to God. See "Supplications (*ad'iya*)," Appendix 3.
8. Patients may want to remember (*dhikr*) the name of God. Some Muslims chant the name of God, which is "Allah" in Arabic, or verses from the Qur'an or repeat the names of God. See Appendix 8 for a list of God's names.
9. Check in with family members about helping their loved one recite the declaration of faith (*shahadah*): "*ash-hadu an la ilaha illa Llah wa ash-hadu anna Muhammadan rasulu Llah*" or "I witness that there is no god but God, and I witness that Muhammad is the Messenger of God." While the dying patient says the *shahadah*, her or his right index finger should be pointing upward.
10. Some families may want to recite in Arabic Qur'an 36 (*Ya-Sin*), or play a recording of this scripture. See "Supplications (*ad'iya*)," Appendix 3. Some

Muslims believe that this *sura* facilitates the ease of passage from this world to the next. Others do not want a recitation of the *sura*. A free recording of this scripture is available on the Internet at http://www.bomb-mp3.com/index.php?search=abdul+rahman+al+sudais+036+surah+yasiin. Pastoral services may have to provide a copy of the Qur'an if the patient or the family does not have one with them. If they are unable to recite the *sura* in Arabic, or if a recording is unavailable, ask if they would like to read an English translation or if they prefer someone else to do it. Some Muslims may be upset if a non-Muslim person tries to read the Qur'an in Arabic, in a transliterated version, or in English, which is why it is important always to ask first. Recitation of *Ya-Sin* takes about 10-20 minutes, depending on the reader's fluency.

11. Play a CD of the Qur'an. Help the family to get a CD from a local mosque or Islamic center or from someone they know. Recordings of the Qur'an are available at various Internet sites, including Islamicity.com, http://www.islamicity.com/mosque/ Qur'an. Have the Qur'an available in Arabic, English, and Urdu. Depending on the ethnicity of the patient population, provide translations in other languages, such as Spanish, French, and German.

12. Know on whom to call for help from local mosques or Islamic centers.

13. Recommend to the family that they get support from their imam or religious leader in preparing the body at the hospital for burial later. Before beginning burial preparations, suggest that the family ask the nurse to remove all medical paraphernalia from the body. Hospital bedside burial preparations include closing the deceased's eyelids, tying closed the mouth (if the family desires), cleaning bodily fluids and substances from the body, straightening

the legs, placing the arms at the side of the body, elevating slightly the body at the head, and covering the body. The deceased patient already should be facing toward Mecca, Saudi Arabia.

14. Give funeral information to the family at the appropriate time.

NOTES

[1] Muhammad Saed Abdul-Rahman, *Tafsir Ibn Kathir Juz' 27 (Part 27): Az-Zariyat 31 to Al-Hadid 29, Part 27* (London: MSA Publication Limited, 2009), 132.

[2] Phone interview with Aysha Saeed, M.D., ABIHM, Hartford, Connecticut, February 2010.

[3] Aziz Sheikh and Abdul Rashid Gatrad, "Death and bereavement: an exploration and a meditation," in *Caring for Muslim Patients*, 2nd ed. Eds. Aziz Sheikh and Abdul Rashid Gatrad (Oxon, United Kingdom: Radcliffe Publishing, 2009), 104.

[4] Helmut Ritter and John O'Kane, *The Ocean of the Soul: Man, the World, and God in the Stories of Farid al-Din*, part I, vol. 69, trans. John O'Kane (Leiden: E.J. Brill, 2003), 190.

[5] Fazlur Rahman, *Health and Medicine in the Islamic Tradition*, (New York: Crossroad Publishing, 1989), 60.

[6] Yahya ibn Sharaf al-Nawawi, *Gardens of the Righteous*, trans. Muhammad Zafrulla Khan (London: Curzon Press, 1989), 173.

## CHAPTER 11

# EUTHANASIA, SUICIDE, AND ASSISTED SUICIDE

Maryam, 85, is in a coma. Fourteen weeks ago, she stopped breathing and suffered heart failure. More than ten minutes passed before paramedics arrived at her home. At the hospital, physicians and nurses got her heart beating in a normal rhythm and put her on a respirator because she could not breathe on her own. However, a CAT-scan established irreversible cessation of all functions of her cerebrum and brain stem. Maryam is brain dead.

She often had told her family that she never wanted to be placed on a respirator or other life-sustaining device. Unfortunately, Maryam had not made an advance healthcare directive or living will. Because of this, and because her husband had died five years earlier, decisions about her healthcare default to her five grown children. Three children think Maryam should be allowed to die naturally. The other two think "pulling the plug" could be tantamount to murder, but the physician assures them otherwise. Maryam is brain dead, he says, and nothing more can be done for her. Continuing the respirator only would prolong her dying. The children agree to have their mother removed from the respirator. Moments later, surrounded by her children, Maryam dies quietly.

## Islamic Perspective on Euthanasia, Suicide, and Assisted Suicide

In the area of medical ethics, discussions about euthanasia, suicide, and assisted suicide often raise more questions than provide answers. One aspect of the debate centers on the use of medication or other methods to deliberately hasten the death of sick, dying patients (called active euthanasia or mercy killing). Others argue that, at the very least, physicians have the right to withhold or withdraw treatment from terminally ill patients. Some call this passive euthanasia (dysthanasia), while others say that any inaction is a decision. Then, there is the question whether mentally competent, terminally ill patients have the right to end their own lives – on their own or with the help of others (suicide or assisted suicide). Moreover, some contend that family members or legal spokespersons have the right to withhold or withdraw treatments if their sick, dying loved ones are unable to do so. Others hold that the grown children of sick, dying patients can challenge their parents' decision to withdraw from life support. Islam, however, "views life as sacred and a 'trust' from Allah; thus, suicide and euthanasia are prohibited."[1] Furthermore, Muslims never hasten or pray for death because they believe that death comes at the decreed hour for their ultimate spiritual benefit. About this, the Prophet Muhammad, says, "None of you should wish for death or for any calamity that befalls you, but should say: 'O Allah! Cause me to live so long as life is better for me, and cause me to die when death is better for me.'"[2] Additionally, "sick people, as indeed healthy ones too, are strongly prohibited from desiring or praying for death, let alone committing suicide; for if a person is good, he may do more good if he lives longer, and if a person is not good, longer life may afford him a chance for conversion. So far as possible, a sick person should not shout of pain or discomfort but try to be of good cheer." [3]

In part, this view is due to the belief that devastating or terminal illness and suffering, like all things, come from God. Moreover, in Islam, the ultimate purpose of any suffering is to increase one's faith. Qur'an 2:153 states: "O you who have attained to faith! Seek aid in steadfast patience and prayer: for, behold, God is with those who are patient in adversity." Islamic tradition says, "When God intends to do good to somebody, He afflicts him with trials."[4] Thus, suffering brings opportunities for reward for Muslims.

Islam also maintains that illness and suffering have a cleansing effect. In Qur'an 2:157, God says, "It is they upon whom their Sustainer's blessings and grace are bestowed, and it is they, they who are on the right path!" Upon visiting a sick person, Prophet Muhammad said, "…Allah removes the sins of a Muslim for his [or her] illness, as fire removes the dross from gold and silver."[5] Another tradition says that "when the Prophet visited a sick person he would say, 'No fear, it [illness] is a catharsis, God willing.'"[6]

## Active and Passive Euthanasia

Withholding nutrition and hydration/withdrawing life-sustaining treatments (passive euthanasia), and using lethal methods (active euthanasia) in order to deliberately hasten the death of terminal patients violates Islamic law and, in fact, is deemed murder. Qur'an 5:32 states, "…if anyone slays a human being – unless it be [in punishment] for murder or for spreading corruption on earth – it shall be as though he had slain all [hu]mankind; whereas, if anyone saves a life, it shall be as though he had saved the lives of all [hu]mankind."

"Modern Islamic *fatwas* (religious legal rulings) do not bother to elaborate on the means through which mercy killing can be executed. These are naturally numerous. Muslim jurists rather view all forms of euthanasia as murder."[7] A patient refusing nutrition or hydration is another matter. (See below). No means for intentionally causing death is permissible, because only God creates life, and death comes by His permission alone. Qur'an 3:145 says, ". . . no human being can die, save by God's leave, at a term pre-ordained."

Sunni scholar Shaykh Al-Qaradawi issued the following ruling (*fatwa*) about euthanasia or mercy killing. It [euthanasia] is "Islamically forbidden for it encompasses a positive role on the part of the physician to end the life of the patient and hasten his death via lethal injection, electric shock, a sharp weapon or any other way. This is an act of killing, and, killing is a major sin and thus forbidden in Islam, the religion of pure mercy."[8]

### Withholding or Withdrawing Treatment

When continuing treatment prolongs the agony of death or does not improve a patient's quality of existence, the elimination of suffering becomes the primary determinant in Islam. In these cases, the patient or legal representative may refuse continuing medical treatment. About this, Islamic jurist Qaradawi says, "… preventing the patient from his [or her] due medication, which is from a medical perspective thought to be useless, this is permissible and sometimes it is even recommended. Thus, the physician can do this for the sake of the patient's comfort and the relief of his family."[9] Significantly, Qaradawi says that such an action is "different from the controversial euthanasia or mercy killing as it does not imply a positive action on the part of the physician; rather, it is some sort of leaving what is not obligatory or recommended, and thus entails no responsibility."[10] It is important to note that if the patient is a child, the parents are responsible for consulting with healthcare professionals, religious leaders, and others in order to make informed decisions about the physical and emotional well-being of the child. Additionally, Reza Mansoor, M.D., cardiologist at Hartford Hospital and assistant clinical professor at the University of Connecticut School of Medicine, Hartford, Conn., says that "stopping medications and even the ventilator in a 'medically futile' situation, as determined by medical personnel, is considered allowable as long as the intention is to give the patient a chance to breathe on his/her own, but if during that period, the person dies, Muslims believe that the death is the will (*qadr*) of God." In such cases, Dr. Mansoor says that before the ventilator would be removed from the patient, his or her family or spokesperson would designate the patient a do-not-intubate, meaning the patient would not be re-instated on the ventilator.[11]

The religious opinion of Islamic jurist Qaradawi also applies to withholding or withdrawing treatment for patients, such as Maryam, the fictitious person described earlier in this chapter. These patients are "medically presumed dead through what is known as brain death … especially when it's clear that the life support machine becomes of no use for the already-dead patient."[12] Jurists allow this action because it is not a variant of euthanasia.

Furthermore, according to the Islamic Medical Association of North America (IMANA), death is established when a person's "cardiopulmonary function has come to a permanent stop" and [when] "the function of the brain, including the brain stem, has come to a permanent stop, even if some other organs may continue to show spontaneous activity."[13]

IMANA also recommends that all Muslims have living wills and advance directives. When death is imminent or coma becomes irreversible, these documents declare a person's end-of-life desire to forgo emergency measures or to appoint a surrogate decision maker. Muslims should consult with family members and attorneys when drafting these legal documents.[14] An Islamic living will and advance directive, which can be adapted to fit the specific needs of patients, is available at the IMANA's website: http://www.isna.net/Leadership/pages/Islamic-Medical-Ethics.aspx/.

Moreover, easing a patient's pain with strong painkillers is permitted. Should this bring about the patient's death, the focus of scrutiny would be on the physician's intention (*niyya*), not the death of the patient. Did the physician purposely end the patient's life, or was the death a result of his/her action intended to alleviate suffering? According to Dr. Mansoor, "medications, such as morphine, can be given for pain and suffering and this may cause earlier death but if the intension is purely for the alleviation of pain and suffering, this is permissible."[15] Muslims believe that only God really knows a person's true intentions.[16] According to Qur'an 40:19, God "... is aware of the [most] stealthy glance, and of all that the hearts would conceal." However, Muslim jurists and legal authorities must perform their temporal duties by determining the motives of crimes.

### Suicide and Assisted Suicide

Islam absolutely forbids suicide. In Qur'an 6:151, God says, "... do not take any human being's life '[the life] which God has declared to be sacred' otherwise than in [the pursuit of] justice ..." Prophet Muhammad warned of dire consequences awaiting those who commit suicide. He declared, "If somebody commits suicide with anything in this world, he will be tortured with that very thing on the Day of Resurrection."[17] Should a patient commit suicide by means of refusing food or hydration, he/she would suffer the same fate in the Hereafter, according to this *hadith*. However, sick people refuse food and hydration all the time because they feel too sick and tired. Here, the *hadith* about the death of Prophet Muhammad is critical – he was forced medicine when he was ill and could not fight back. When he came to for a while, he punished those who forced him by forcing them to take the medicine.[18]

The *shari'a* also prohibits assisted suicide. Should a physician prescribe, but not administer, life-ending medications that a patient uses to commit suicide, jurists say it would be the same as if that physician himself had murdered that patient. The same ruling applies to anyone helping another to end his/her life.[19] About this, the members of the European Council for Fatwa and Research issued the following ruling: "It is unlawful for the patient to kill himself (or herself) and it is unlawful for somebody else to kill him (or her) even if he (or she) is given leave to kill him (or her). The former case will be suicide and the latter will be aggression against the other by killing him [or her] for his [or her] permission does not render the unlawful act lawful. The patient does not possess his [or her] own soul to permit somebody else to take it."[20]

### Summary

1. Withholding and withdrawing life-sustaining treatments to hasten early death violates Islamic law.

2. Using lethal means to cause early death violates Islamic law.
3. Suicide and assisted suicide violate Islamic law.
4. However, refusing, withdrawing, or withholding medical life-support treatments that do not improve the quality of existence of terminally ill or brain-dead patients is permitted in Islamic law.
5. Administering pain relief that ultimately shortens life is permitted provided the intention is not to end the life of the patient.

## PRACTICAL STEPS FOR CARING FOR MUSLIM PATIENTS

Life is sacred in Islam. However, when death is inevitable, under certain conditions, the patient or his/her legal representative may refuse life-sustaining medical treatment. Islam prohibits suicide, assisted suicide, and active or passive euthanasia. Any discussions about the medical condition of an unconscious patient should take place away from that patient.

### Before Talking with the Family

1. See the "Islamic Perspective on Euthanasia, Suicide, and Assisted Suicide" section.
2. Talk with physicians and nurses about the patient's medical situation and mental state.
3. Become familiar with state laws and hospital protocol for withdrawing life-support treatments.
4. Understand hospital guidelines for releasing the body of a deceased patient.
5. Have available funeral- and burial-planning information. See "Practical Steps at Death of a Muslim Patient," Appendix 1.

### Once with the Family

1. Encourage the family to contact their imam or religious leader for support.
2. Assess and provide support for the family's physical, emotional, and spiritual needs.
3. Ask the physician to explain to the family, in your presence, the patient's medical state.
4. Ask the family about their cultural and faith beliefs concerning the removal of life-support.
5. Help the family understand that in Islam, the removal of life support in order not to prolong the agony of death when death is inevitable is permissible.
6. Often families feel guilty about removing life support. Assure the family that in Islam, God alone determines the time of death, that according to the physician's assessment, nothing more can be done for the patient.
7. Ask if the family would like to make supplication (*du'a*) for the dying (or dead) loved one or if they prefer that a hospital worker read the English translation of a specific Qur'anic verse (*aya*). Be aware that some Muslims are offended if non-Muslims read the Qur'an. Ask first. Never invoke the name of Jesus in prayers; this is offensive to Muslims, who pray only to God. See "Supplications (*ad'iya*)," Appendix 3.
8. Some Muslims may want to repeat (*dhikr*) the names of God. See Appendix 8 for a list of God's names.
9. Encourage the family to make remembrance (*dhikr*) of God's name(s) while the loved one is alive (even though unconscious) and after the patient dies. Many Muslims believe that an unconscious person and a recently deceased person can hear.
10. If the family follows the practice of reciting Qur'an 36 (*Ya-Sin*) for the

dying and deceased patient, provide them with a copy of this scripture, or play a recording of it. See Appendix 3. A free Internet recording of the sura is available at http://www.bomb-mp3.com/index.php?search=abdul+rahman+al+sudais+036+surah+yasiin.

11. Ask the family if they would like to help their loved one recite the declaration of faith (*shahadah*). The shahadah: "*ash-hadu an la ilaha illa Llah wa ash-hadu anna Muhammadan rasulu Llah*" or "I witness that there is no god but God, and I witness that Muhammad is the Messenger of God." A family member, the family's imam or religious leader should recite the *shahadah* in the right ear of the deceased person.

12. Shortly before the death of the patient, suggest that the family call their imam or religious leader for support in preparing the body for burial.

13. Provide the family with contact information for Muslim funeral homes, Islamic centers and mosques that follow Islamic rituals for preparing a body for burial.

NOTES

[1] Aziz Sheikh and Abdul Rashid Gatrad, "Death and bereavement: an exploration and a meditation," in *Caring for Muslim Patients*, 2nd ed. Eds. Aziz Sheikh and Abdul Rashid Gatrad (Oxon, United Kingdom: Radcliffe Publishing, 2009), 104.

[2] Abu Dawud 3102, Bukhan 70.19.575, in Ruqaiyyah Waris Maqsood, *Islam*, 2nd ed. (Oxford, England: Heinemann Educational Publishers, 1995), 134.

[3] Fazlur Rahman, *Health and Medicine in the Islamic Tradition*, (New York: Crossroad Publishing, 1989), 60.

[4] *Sahih Bukhari, hadith* 546, in *Abdul Sachedina, Islamic Biomedical Ethics: Principles and Applications* (Oxford: Oxford University Press, 2009), 93.

[5] Abu Dawud 3086, in Raqaiyyah Waris Maqsood, *After Death, Life! Thoughts to alleviate the Grief of all Muslims facing Death and Bereavement* (Lahore: Talha Publication, 2001), 105.

[6] Rahman, 59.

[7] Vardit Rispler-Chaim, *Islamic Medical Ethics in the Twentieth Century* (Leiden: E.J. Brill, 1993), 95.

[8] Yusuf Al-Qaradawi, "Islam's Stance on Euthanasia," Islamonline.net fatwa databank of Qaradawi, http://www.islamonline.net/servlet/Satellite?pagename=IslamOnline-English-Ask_Scholar/FatwaE/FatwaE&cid=1119503544774. Accessed 20 December 2009.

[9] Ibid.

[10] Ibid.

[11] From email correspondence with Reza Mansoor, M.D., cardiologist at Hartford Hospital and assistant clinical professor at the University of Connecticut School of Medicine, Hartford, Connecticut, May 1, 2011.

[12] Ibid.

[13] IMANA Ethics Committee, "Islamic Medical Ethics," available at the web site of the Islamic Society of North America, http://www.isna.net/Leadership/pages/Islamic-Medical-Ethics.aspx. Accessed 19 February 2010.

[14] Islamic Society of North America (ISNA), http://www.isna.net/Leadership/pages/Islamic-Medical-Ethics.aspx. Accessed 8 January 2010.

[15] Email correspondence from Reza Mansoor, M.D., May 1, 2011.

[16] Hassan Hathout, *Reading the Muslim Mind* (Plainfield, IN: American Trust Publications, 1995), 134-35.

[17] Muhammad ibn Ismail al-Bukhari, *Sahih Bukhari,* Volume 8, Book 73, Number 73, narrated by Thabit bin Ad-Dahhak, one of the companions who gave the pledge of

allegiance to the Prophet underneath the tree (Al-Hudaibiya). (*Sahih Bukhari,* 8:73:73 [see also 2:23:445, 2:23:446, 8:73:126, 8:78:647]).

[18] Muhammad ibn Ismail al-Bukhari, *Sahih Bukhari,* Volume 9, Book 83, Number 25, "Blood Money (*Ad-Diyat*)," University of Southern California *ahadith* database: http://www.usc.edu/schools/college/crcc/engagement/resources/texts/muslim/hadith/bukhari/083.sbt.html. Accessed 9 April 2010.

[19] European Council for Fatwa and Research at http://www.islamonline.net/servlet/Satellite?pagename=IslamOnline-English-Ask_Scholar/FatwaE/FatwaE&cid=1119503549272. Accessed 21 November 2009

[20] Ibid.

# CHAPTER 12

# FERTILITY REGULATION

Tahera and her husband have five children. He wants to have another child, but she does not; they are in difficult financial straits. She has told him that having another baby would cause undue hardship on the children they already have and that she wants to take birth-control pills. Her husband disagreed, saying, "God will provide." Tahera consulted with her imam (religious leader), who told her that under Islamic law birth control requires consensual spousal agreement. The imam meets with Tahera's husband and provides him with reports of the sayings of Prophet Muhammad (*hadith*, sg. /*ahadith*, pl.) and legal opinions (*fatwas*) of the leading jurists in support of contraception.

## Islamic Perspective on Fertility Regulation

Islamic jurists turn to the *ahadith*, the second source of law, to determine the permissibility of contraception. This is because the highest and most respected source of guidance in Islam, the Qur'an, does not speak directly to the issue. Most often cited are the *ahadith* of the companions of Prophet Muhammad. One well-known *hadith* comes from the collection *Sahih Muslim*. In it, a companion of Prophet Muhammad states: "'We practiced coitus interruptus ['*azl* ] during the time of the Messenger of Allah (peace be upon him). He came to know about it, but he did not prohibit it.'"[1] Because of this *hadith* and other trusted *ahadith*, Islamic jurists reason (*qiyas*) consensually (*ijma*) that Prophet Muhammad verbally or tacitly approved the practice of contraception by Muslims.[2] Thus, they say, contraception is not forbidden; however, they do not grant categorical approval.[3] The issue of contraception is relevant only to married heterosexual couples. Islam forbids intercourse outside of marriage.

Muslim women, in agreement with their husbands, may prevent pregnancy using hormone-releasing skin patches, intrauterine devices (IUDs), birth-control pills, and other options, so long as the method does not cause abortion or sterility. In Islam, most jurists frown upon any procedure that results in sterility (partial or full hysterectomy, tubal ligation, or vasectomy), unless done for medical reasons. The only exception applies to "women with a reasonable number of children who are approaching the end of their reproductive life."[4] In such cases, both spouses must agree upon the procedure.[5]

Muslim husbands may not force their wives to practice contraception or to have children. In the *ahadith* collection of Imam Ahmad bin Hanbal, Prophet Muhammad says, ". . . contraception requires the consent of the wife because she has a right both to sexual enjoyment and to decide whether or not she wants a child."[6] Furthermore, "in Islam the wife has the inalienable right to sexual satisfaction, and the Prophet is reported to have granted divorce to a woman on grounds of her husband's impotency when she complained."[7]

A leading Sunni jurist Shaykh Yusuf Qaradawi approves of contraception for two reasons. His opinion (*fatwa*) is as follows.[8]

1. "The first valid reason for employing contraception is the fear that the pregnancy or delivery might endanger the life or health of the mother; past experience, or the opinion of a reliable physician, are the guides in determining this possibility. Allah Ta'ala says: '...And do not be cast into ruin by your own hands...' [2:195]."
2. "Another reason is the fear that the burden of children may straiten [debilitate] the family's circumstances so much that one might accept or do something *haram* [religiously forbidden] to satisfy their needs. Allah says: '... Allah desires ease for you, and He does not desire hardship for you...' [2:185]."

The preeminent Shia jurist Ali Sistani approves contraception, but with a qualifier. He said, "It is permissible for a woman to use contraceptives (the pill) to prevent pregnancy provided it does not harm her health in a serious manner, irrespective of whether or not the husband has agreed to it."[9]

The position of the Islamic Medical Association of North America (IMANA) on contraception is as follows:

> For married couples, contraception for several reasons, including health of the mother, social or economic reasons, etc., is permitted, provided that it is practiced by mutual agreement of the husband and wife and that the method used is reversible and not harmful. Withdrawal, prophylactics, birth control pills, and other hormonal methods are allowed. Contraceptive methods which can lead to abortion are not allowed."[10]

### Summary

1. Most Islamic jurists permit contraceptive practices for the prevention of pregnancy, excluding any method that causes abortion. They also prohibit sterilization as a method of contraception unless it protects a woman's health and life or if a woman with children is nearing menopause. Any sterilization procedure requires a husband's approval.
2. The IMANA position is that contraception for the "health of the mother, social or economic reasons" is permissible, but not for purposes of abortion, sterility, or to do harm. Both spouses must agree to it.
3. Shia jurist Ali Sistani approves contraception, but only for the prevention of pregnancy, and only so long as it does not harm the woman. The husband's approval, he says, is not required.
4. Sunni jurist Shaykh Yusuf Qaradawi permits contraception in cases where pregnancy would endanger the health or life of a woman and in situations where more children would be economically damaging to the family.

## PRACTICAL STEPS FOR CARING FOR MUSLIM PATIENTS

Muslim women may use birth control to prevent pregnancy so long as it does not cause abortion or sterility, and so long as the husband agrees. Where there is disagreement, one or both spouses may ask the chaplain or healthcare worker to mediate or provide information that could help them resolve the issue amicably. Additionally, the need for contraception may be for health reasons, and the patient and her husband may be struggling with the reality of having no more children.

**Before Talking with the Patient or Her Husband**

1. Read the "Fertility Regulation" chapter.
2. Talk with the patient's healthcare providers for an assessment of the patient's physical and mental states. Ask them also about the husband's emotional state. Is he supportive or opposed to contraception?

**Once at the Bedside of the Patient or with her Husband**

1. Get an understanding of why the patient and her husband want to prevent pregnancy. Is it for health or financial reasons, for example?
2. Support the patient's decision not to have another child at this time. If it is a lifetime decision because of health issues, help them process the decision.
3. Chaplains or other healthcare workers may provide supplication (*du'a*) to God, if the family desires. See "Supplications (*ad'iya*)," Appendix 3. Some Muslims may be comfortable or offended with the reading of the Qur'an by a non-Muslim. Ask first. Never invoke the name of Jesus in prayers; this is offensive to Muslims, who pray only to God.
4. Some Muslims may want to repeat (*dhikr*) the names of God. See Appendix 8 for a list of God's names.

NOTES

[1] Yusuf al-Qaradawi, The Lawful, *The Lawful and the Prohibited in Islam,* trans. Kamal El-Helbawy, M. Moinuddin Siddiqui, Syed Shukry (Indianapolis, IN: American Trust Publications, 1982), 198.

[2] Riffat Hassan, "Is Family Planning Permitted in Islam?" in *Muslim Women Scholar-activists in North America,* ed. Giesla Webb (Syracuse, NY: Syracuse University Press, 2000), 232.

[3] Zulie Sachedina, "Islam, Procreation and the Law," *International Family Planning Perspectives* 16, No. 3 (Sept. 1990): 108-9.

[4] Hasan Hathout, *Reading the Muslim Mind* (Plainfield, IN: American Trust Publications, 1995), 125.

[5] Ibid.

[6] Qaradawi, *The Lawful,* 201.

[7] Fazlur Rahman, *Health and Medicine in the Islamic Tradition,* (New York: Crossroad Publishing, 1989), 121.

[8] Ibid., 199-200.

[9] Ali Sistani (No. 407), *A Code of Practice for Muslims in the West,* trans. Sayyid Muhammad Rizvi (London, England: Imam Ali Foundation, 1999), 208.

[10] IMANA Ethics Committee, "Islamic Medical Ethics," available at the website of the Islamic Society of North America, http://www.isna.net/Leadership/pages/Islamic-Medical-Ethics.aspx. Accessed 19 February 2010.

## CHAPTER 13

# INFERTILITY TREATMENT

Hamid and Aziza got married in their late thirties. They immediately started planning for children, but it soon became clear that Aziza had fertility problems. To help her conceive, doctors tried artificial insemination using Hamid's sperm, but it did not work. They next tried in-vitro fertilization (her ovum fertilized outside the uterus with Hamid's sperm and implanted into her womb), but that did not work either. As a last resort, doctors suggest using Hamid's sperm to fertilize another woman's ovum, which then would be implanted in Aziza's womb. The couple refuses this on religious grounds and resign themselves to remaining childless.

### Islamic Perspective on Infertility Treatment

Marriage is strongly encouraged in Islam. In a saying (*hadith*) of Prophet Muhammad, he said, "Marriage is my tradition. He who rejects my tradition is not of me."[1] Muslims believe that children are gifts from God. According to Qur'an 16:72, "And God has given you mates of your own kind and has given you, through your mates, children and children's children, and has provided for you sustenance out of the good things of life." However, if a husband and wife cannot conceive on their own, they may seek fertility treatment.

Muslim jurists permit fertility treatments based on the following tenets of Islam.

- "Islamic law acknowledges that pregnancy can sometimes occur other than by direct sexual contact, i.e., without penetration. The child born though indirect/artificial insemination is therefore legitimate."[2]
- "Bringing about pregnancy by means other than direct sexual contact is not perceived as interference in the Creator's acts, nor as contesting God's wish and decree. On the contrary: Islam desires that [hu]mankind be happy. Artificial insemination was made possible through knowledge which God has provided. Medicine alone is not capable of producing an egg or semen. It can only improve the way the two unite, after God has created them."[3]

There are strict guidelines about assisted reproduction, however.

Islamic law says that a heterosexual couple must be contractually married in order to participate in assisted reproduction. "Islam would not permit the union of genes of a male and a female who are not husband and wife, because this would, it appears, constitute adultery under Islamic law. For under Islamic law, adultery does not mean merely the physical sexual intercourse between an unmarried couple but also refers to a situation where the descent of a child is mixed up …"[4] Furthermore, both spouses must be living. A deceased husband's sperm or a wife's ovum cannot be used in any form of artificial insemination by the living spouse after the death of the other spouse. In Islam, marriage ends at death.[5]

Furthermore, Islamic law forbids gestational surrogacy (contracting with another woman to carry a couple's biological child) – because women must birth their own offspring and because family lineage must be protected. "Children have the right to be born through a legitimate union, with full knowledge of their parentage... [and] have the right to a good name, to be suckled, educated and, above all, to have a loving and caring environment in which they may thrive to fulfill their Allah given potential." [6]

Muslim women must bear their own children because Qur'an 58:2 says, "...none are their mothers save those who gave them birth..." If a couple ignores the prohibition and proceeds with surrogacy to have a baby, "it is the consensus of Islamic scholars that the birth mother is the 'real' mother." [7]

Some childless couples turn to adopting (*tabanna*) and fostering (*nafaqah*) of a child.

In Islam, however, legally adopting is forbidden. The basis for this prohibition stems from the primary source of Islamic law, the Qur'an. In Qur'an 4:5, God says, "And do not entrust to those who are weak of judgment the possessions which God has placed in your charge for [their] support; but let them have their sustenance therefrom, and clothe them, and speak unto them in a kindly way." Furthermore, Qur'an 33:5 says, "...call them by their [real] fathers' names: this is more equitable in the sight of God..." Islam wants what is best for orphaned children. The prohibition against adopting protects an orphaned child's birth identity and lineage (*nasab*).[8] Inheritance, marriage, and other social conventions in Islam are based on blood relationship. Before Islam, Arab tribes gained dominance by adopting children, usually males, and grown men and slaves from other tribes in order to eradicate the lineage of their opponents. Nevertheless, after the revelation of Qur'an 4:5, the practice of adopting ended.

Fostering a child is a legal obligation for male relatives in Islam. "A fatherless child is considered an orphan (*yatim*) even if his or her mother is still living. In most religious schools of law, a needy orphan has the right to maintenance from a male relative even if the mother retains custody (*hadanah*)."[9] The secondary source of Islamic law, the words and deeds of Prophet Muhammad (*hadith*, sg./*ahadith*, pl.), and, in particular, the following *hadith*, confirms the permissibility of *nafaqah*. "Abu Huraira reported that Allah's Messenger (may peace be upon him) said: 'One who looks after the orphan whether he is his relative or not, I and he would be together in Paradise like this,' and Malik (explained it) with the gesture by drawing his index finger and middle finger close together."[10] After Prophet Muhammad was orphaned at an early age, his grandfather, Abd al-Muttalib, became his guardian (*waliyah*) and then his uncle, Abu Talib.

## Summary

1. Artificial insemination: Using the husband's sperm to fertilize his wife's ovum in the uterus is allowed in Islamic law.
2. In vitro fertilization (IVF): Islamic law permits fertilizing several of the wife's ova outside her womb by her husband's sperm and transferring them into the woman's uterus.
3. Gestational surrogacy or donation: Islamic law prohibits employing another's ova or sperm or uterus for procreation purposes. It is fornication, because only contractually married heterosexual couples are allowed to procreate.

## PRACTICAL STEPS FOR CARING FOR MUSLIM PATIENTS

In Islam, having children is exclusive to heterosexual marriage. If a husband and wife are unable to conceive, they may seek help from medical science, but always in accordance with Islamic law.

### BEFORE TALKING WITH THE PATIENT AND HER HUSBAND

1. Read the "Infertility Treatment" chapter.
2. Ask the patient's physician and nurses about the patient's infertility situation, about her feelings on the issue, and check with them about her husband's feelings, too.

### ONCE AT THE BEDSIDE OF THE PATIENT OR WITH HER HUSBAND

1. Encourage the patient and her husband to get support from their religious leader.
2. Support the couple's decision to seek infertility treatment that aligns with their beliefs and cultural persuasions.
3. Chaplains or other healthcare workers may want to provide supplication (*du'a*) to God, if the family desires. See "Supplications (*ad'iya*)," Appendix 3. Ask if the couple wants a chaplain or healthcare worker to read the Qur'anic scripture in English or if they prefer to recite the Qur'an. Some Muslims may be offended if a non-Muslim reads the Qur'an. Never invoke the name of Jesus in prayers; this is offensive to Muslims. Muslims pray only to God.

NOTES

[1] Shahid Athar, *Sex Education: An Islamic Perspective* (South Elgin, IL: KAZI Publications, 1995), 14.

[2] Vardit Rispler-Chaim, *Islamic Medical Ethics in the Twentieth Century* (Leiden: E.J. Brill, 1993), 20.

[3] Ibid., 21.

[4] Fazlur Rahman, *Health and Medicine in the Islamic Tradition*, (New York: Crossroad Publishing, 1989), 107.

[5] Shahid Athar, "Islamic Medical Ethics," *Islamic Horizons* (January / February 2002): 41.

[6] Abdul Rashid Gatrad and Aziz Sheikh, "Birth Customs: meaning and significance," in *Caring for Muslim Patients*, 2nd ed. Eds. Aziz Sheikh and Abdul Rashid Gatrad (Oxon, United Kingdom: Radcliffe Publishing, 2009), 68.

[7] Hossam E. Fadel, "The Islamic Viewpoint on New Assisted Reproductive Technologies," 30 *Fordham Urban Law Journal* 147 (November 2002): 154.

[8] Phone interview with Aminah Assilmi (b. 1945 / d. 2010) a broadcast journalist and former director of the International Union of Muslim Women.

[9] Ingrid Mattson, "Adopting Children," *Islamic Horizons*, (January/February 2008) http://www.isnawebpaper.com/webpapers/isna0801/multi/index.html. Accessed 10 April 2010.

[10] Muslim ibn al-Hajjaj, *Sahih Muslim*, Volume 9, Book 42, Number 7108, University of Southern California *ahadith* database: http://www.usc.edu/schools/college/crcc/engagement/resources/texts/muslim/hadith/muslim/042.smt.html. Accessed 9 April 2010.

## CHAPTER 14

# ORGAN TRANSPLANTATION

Three-year-old Farah was crying and had a fever. Her mother Salima thought that Farah had the flu, but when the toddler stopped urinating, she took her to the doctor. It turned out to be severe hyperoxaluria, a rare disorder that causes liver and kidney failure. Immediately, the physician admitted Farah to a hospital pediatric intensive care and put her on dialysis and hemodialysis. Three weeks later, the physician told Farah's parents that the toddler's liver and kidneys were failing fast, that she needed transplants, and that those organs had just become available from a non-Muslim child who had died in a car accident a few hours earlier.

As compatible donor organs are rare (there are more than 100,000 people in the U.S. on waiting lists), many parents would rejoice at such news. Farah's did not. Even though they were aware that Farah would die without the organ transplants, they hesitated. They were from Pakistan, where Muslim jurists advise against organ donation.[1]

Knowing that Farah's life depends on her parents' decision, the transplant team, a local imam (religious leader), and social worker provided the couple with medical and religious information. This enabled them to decide in favor of the organ transplants, while still doing what they considered religiously correct.

## Islamic Perspective on Organ Transplantation

Although nothing in the Qur'an or the actions and words of Prophet Muhammad (*Sunna*) prohibits organ transplant (as it did not exist in the early Islam), differences of opinion abound. Legal opinions of Islamic jurists (*fatwas*), which uphold the principles of the Qur'an and *Sunna*, vary according to locale. Jurists from Arab countries generally permit organ transplant. Those from South Asia often forbid it, saying it desecrates the donor's body. They cite a report (*hadith*, sg./*ahadith*, pl.) of the Prophet Muhammad that warns "breaking the bones of the dead is as offensive as breaking the bones of the living."[2] Jurists from the Indian subcontinent concur with this prohibition, but for slightly different reasons. They maintain that "since life is a 'trust', one has no right to 'donate' any part of one's body to someone else."[3] Others say that the physical body must remain intact in order to be raised whole from the dead on the Day of Resurrection. While bodily resurrection is a fundamental belief in Islam, the idea that the body must remain intact for this to occur is not based on the Qur'an. In fact, God says in Qur'an 75:3-4, "Does man think that We cannot [resurrect him and] bring his bones together again? Yea indeed, We are able to make whole his very finger-tips!" No one knows at what age the body will be resurrected. Some conjecture that "we will either gain or decrease in years in the Garden so as to be at the median age."[4]

Despite these prohibitions, an increasing number of Muslims believe that organ donation is permissible, and even desirable. Their belief is based on the Islamic doctrine that "necessity allows the prohibited" and lives must be saved.[5] According to Qur'an 5:32, "If anyone saves a life, it shall be as though he had saved the lives of all [hu]mankind." Furthermore, there is the Islamic doctrine that states that "the needs of a living human have priority over those of a dead one." This doctrine, according to Fazlur Rahman, an Islamic scholar, comes from various *ahadith* that "say that expensive shrouds should not be provided to the dead because living people need cloth more than the dead. According to the Shafi'i School, "if a pregnant woman is dying, her baby should be extracted from her womb if it has a good chance of survival."[6]

An additional point of doctrine is that Muslims, as a community, have collective responsibilities, such as sharing wealth (almsgiving and charity). However, not every member of the community must fulfill these responsibilities. When an individual or group fulfills these responsibilities, they are considered to be fulfilled by all. Conversely, if neglected by the community as a whole, each individual "bears the moral responsibility for their failure as a group."[7]

Many highly respected Islamic institutions have declared organ donation as an act of merit and, in certain situations, an obligation. These institutions are the Shariah Academy of the Organization of Islamic Conference (representing all Muslim countries); the Grand Ulema Council of Saudi Arabia; the Iranian Religious Authority; and the Al-Azhar Academy of Egypt. "Even the Guardian Council, the Islamic Republic's constitutional overseeing body, which is dominated by the most conservative *mullahs* [male religious teachers or leaders], has recently pronounced an edict allowing organ transplants from dead or brain-dead people."[8]

Additionally, the Muslim Law (*shari'a*) Council U.K. in 1995 issued a *fatwa* in support of organ transplantation. The council said that organ transplantation is a "means of alleviating pain or saving life on the basis of the rules of the Shariah [sic]; Muslims may carry donor cards; and the next of kin of a dead person (in the absence of a card or an expressed wish to donate their organs) may give permission to obtain organs from the body to save other people's lives."[9]

> Furthermore, the Islamic Code of Medical Ethics states: The individual patient is the collective responsibility of Society, that has to ensure his health needs by any means inflicting no harm on others. This comprises the donation of body fluids and organs.... This is another *fard kifaya*, a duty that donors fulfill on behalf of society.[10]

Many Muslim jurists compare the sharing of organs to the sharing of wealth. Both are from God, and God says that wealth should be shared with others. "... and give them [their share] of the wealth of God which He has given you." (Qur'an 24:33), and, ". . . [b]elieve in God and His Apostle, and spend on others out of that of which He has made you trustees: for, those of you who have attained to faith and who spend freely [in God's cause] shall have a great reward." (Qur'an 57:7)

Shia scholar Ali Sistani says, "As far as donating an organ from a living person to the body of another person is concerned, there is no problem in it if it does not entail a serious harm to the donar [sic]."[11] A donated "organ extracted from the body is ritually impure (*najis*), irrespective of whether it came from a Muslim or non-Muslim." Nevertheless, "when it becomes ... part of a Muslim's body ..., it becomes *tahir* [ritually pure]."[12]

The following secular rules, regulations, and conditions of organ transplants align with Islamic principles.

• Consent to donate organs is required by law. Sane and sound adults may freely give consent by registering with state-run donor agencies, by designating the decision to donate on a driver's license, by signing and carrying a donor card, or by noting the intention to donate an organ(s) in a legal will.
• Where no consent is given before death, approval may come from the deceased person's next of kin provided that he/she is legally and ethically able to do so and that the deceased had not indicated that he/she did not want to donate organs.
• After medical authorities establish a person's death, organs may be donated. The Islamic Medical Association of North America (IMANA) says death occurs when "cardiopulmonary function has come to a permanent stop" and [when] "the function of the brain, including the brain stem, has come to a permanent stop, even if some other organs may continue to show spontaneous activity."[13]

## Summary

Most Islamic jurists approve of human organ transplants for the following reasons.
1. A living person donating an organ is permitted so long as the donor is not seriously harmed.
2. Donated organs, whether from a Muslim or non-Muslim, are ritually pure if implanted into the body of a Muslim.
3. Desecrating the body of a deceased person is strictly forbidden in Islam;

however, medical procedures that improve or save lives carry the greater weight of the law. Respecting both life and the dignity of the dead is obligatory for all Muslims.

4. The Islamic doctrine "necessity allows the prohibited" applies to organ transplants from both living and deceased persons.

5. Organ transplantation embodies the Qur'anic precept of whoever saves a life, saves all of humankind. Organ transplants are a gift of life.

6. In the Qur'an, God enjoins humankind to spend of what He has bestowed upon them, including organ donations, according to Shaykh Qaradawi.

7. Muslims have an individual and collective duty to eliminate the suffering of creation.

## PRACTICAL STEPS FOR CARING FOR MUSLIM PATIENTS

Saving lives by donating organs takes precedence over cultural sensitivities, according to most Islamic jurists. The chaplain or other healthcare worker should be aware of these opinions, but their primary responsibility is to support the wishes and needs of the patient's family.

### Before Talking with the Dying Patient or the Family

1. Read the "Islamic Perspective on Organ Transplant" section.
2. Check with the physician and nurses about the patient's cause of death, and ask about the family's mindset toward organ donation.

### Once with the Dying/Deceased Patient's Family

1. Encourage the family of the dying deceased to contact their imam or religious leader for support.

2. For families hesitant about organ donation, the chaplain or other healthcare worker may share information provided above about the benefits of doing so for the recipient and their loved one, if doing so is in line with hospital guidelines.
3. If the family desires, a chaplain or healthcare worker may make supplication (*du'a*) to God. See "Supplications (*ad'iya*)," Appendix 3. Make sure the family is comfortable with a non-Muslim reading the English translation of the Qur'an. Some Muslims consider this disrespectful. They may want to recite the Qur'an themselves. Have available Qur'an 36 (*Ya-Sin*) for those Muslims preferring this scripture. Never invoke the name of Jesus in prayers; this is offensive to Muslims. Muslims pray only to God.

---

NOTES

[1] A.R. Gatrad, "Muslim customs surrounding death, bereavement, post-mortem examinations, and organ transplants," *British Medical Journal* 309 (20 August 1994): 521-3.

[2] Gerrie ter Haar and Yoshio Tsuruoka, *Religion and Society: An Agenda for the 21st Century* (Vol. 5, *International Studies in Religion and Society*) (Leiden: E.J. Brill, 2007), 50.

[3] Aziz Sheikh and Abdul Rashid Gatrad, "Death and bereavement: an exploration and a meditation," in *Caring for Muslim Patients*, 2nd ed. Eds. Aziz Sheikh and Abdul Rashid Gatrad (Oxon, United Kingdom: Radcliffe Publishing, 2009), 111.

[4] Jane I. Smith and Yuonne Yazbeck Haddad, *The Islamic Understanding of Death and Resurrection* (New York: Oxford University Press, 2002), 132.

[5] Sheikh and Gatrad, ibid.

[6] Fazlur Rahman, *Health and Medicine in the Islamic Tradition*, (New York: Crossroad Publishing, 1989),141-42.

[7] Umar Faruq Abd-Allah, ibid. "Living Islam with Purpose" (Nawawi Foundation Paper, 2007), 3, http://www.nawawi.org/downloads/article6.pdf. Accessed 20 November 2009.

[8] Hormoz Ebrahimnejad, "Religion and Medicine in Iran: From Relationship to Dissociation," *British Journal for the History of Science* xl (2002): 16.

[9] NHA Islam and Organ Donor booklet.

[10] International Organization of Islamic Medicine, *Islamic Code of Medical Ethics,* [Kuwait]: International Organization of Islamic Medicine, 1981, quoted in Robert M. Veatch, *Transplantation Ethics* (Washington, D.C.: Georgetown University Press, 2000), 9-10.

[11] Ali Sistani, *A Code of Practice for Muslims in the West,* trans. Sayyid Muhammad Rizvi (London, England: Imam Ali Foundation, 1999), 194.

[12] Ibid. Note: Some Islamic schools of law consider death as defiling; therefore, organs from dead bodies are defiled and could cause donor recipients to become impure.

[13] IMANA Ethics Committee. "Islamic Medical Ethics," available at Islamic Society of North America, http://www.isna.net/Leadership/pages/Islamic-Medical-Ethics.aspx. Accessed 19 February 2010.

## CHAPTER 15

# STEM CELL RESEARCH

After trying to conceive a baby for several years, a Muslim couple decides to try in vitro fertilization. This procedure combines the husband's sperm and wife's ova to grow in a laboratory several fertilized ova of which one or more are implanted into the wife's womb. Any additional fertilized embryos may be frozen and used at another time or may be discarded. In the case of this Muslim couple, after the birth of twins (boy and girl), they decide not to have more children. They donate their remaining embryos to stem cell research.

### Islamic Perspective on Stem Cell Research

Much of the potential and most of the debate about stem cell research centers on the theory that replacement hearts, livers, or virtually any specialized human cell could be grown from human embryonic stem cells (hESCs). At the core of the debate are two potentially conflicting Islamic principles: the duty to respect human life and the duty to reduce human suffering.

This issue raises major ethical questions among Islamic jurists, who question the moral status of un-implanted embryos. Are they human beings? Is it ethical to use them for biomedical research? What sources of hESCs are permissible and which are prohibited? Although there are no Qur'anic injunctions or reports of the words and actions (*hadith*, sg./*ahadith*, pl.) of the Prophet Muhammad that specifically address these questions, jurists have handed down various religious legal opinions (*fatwas*). These fatwas are based on the principles of the Qur'an and the actions and words of Prophet Muhammad (*Sunna*).

Generally, most jurists agree that un-implanted embryos do not represent human life because they cannot grow into human beings. In taking this view, they "seem to maintain a moral distinction between an embryo that is already implanted and developing in the uterus and 'surplus' or 'spare' embryos from IVF.[1]

This is because, although the Qur'an and *ahadith* do not state precisely when human life begins, Islamic jurists think it occurs when the spirit (*ruh*) of God is breathed into the body of the fetus (also referred to in Islamic law as personhood or ensoulment). According to Qur'an 32:6-9, "…the Almighty, the Dispenser of Grace … begins the creation of [the human] out of clay; then He causes [the human] to be begotten out of the essence of a humble fluid; and then He forms [the human] in accordance with what [the human] is meant to be, and breathes into [the human] of His spirit …"

This Qur'anic scripture differentiates biological life, which begins at fertilization, from human life and confers moral status on the fetus. Ensoulment, therefore, represents the "beginning of legally recognized personhood."[2] However, Muslim jurists differ on the timing of ensoulment – 40 days after fertilization or after 120 days.[3] Others place the timing even earlier. Each interpretation is based on the following hadith of Prophet Muhammad:

> ...[E]very one of you is collected in the womb of his mother for the first forty days, and then he becomes a clot for another forty days, and then a piece of flesh for another forty days. Then Allah sends an angel to write four words: He writes his deeds, time of his death, means of his livelihood, and whether he will be wretched or blessed (in religion). Then the soul is breathed into his body."[4]

### Is it Ethical to Destroy Embryos?

Because most Islamic jurists consider un-implanted laboratory embryos to be "biological," organic nonhuman life, "they do not see any moral problem in using frozen embryos for biomedical research"[5] that could lead to new treatments for incurable diseases (e.g., Parkinson's, Alzheimer's, diabetes, and spinal cord injuries).

In fact, these jurists permit the use of hESCs for biomedical research, and consider it a collective moral obligation (*fard kifaya*) on the world's Muslim community.[6] This tenet derives from a *hadith* of Prophet Muhammad that says, "Allah has sent down both the disease and the cure, and He has appointed a cure for every disease, so treat yourselves medically, but use nothing unlawful."[7] In principle, actions are permissible unless prohibited explicitly or contradict established principles of Islamic law.[8]

### What are the Restrictions?

Islamic jurists have established permissible and prohibited sources of stem cells. However, this is not a license to use human embryos "as a product or as a means to an end."[9] The Muslim World League's Islamic Jurisprudence Council issued a *fatwa* (religious opinion) at a conference in December of 2003 in Mecca, Saudi Arabia, about the permissible and prohibited sources of embryonic stem cells. The ruling states that permissible sources are "spontaneously aborted embryos or those aborted for a legally acceptable cause and with the permission of the parents; [and] excess fertilized eggs produced during the course of IVF and donated by the parents with assurance that they are not to be used to produce an illegal pregnancy."[10] Conversely, prohibited sources of stem cells are "intentionally aborted fetuses (abortion without a legal medical reason); intentional fertilization between a donated ovum and sperm; and therapeutic cloning."[11]

### Summary

1. Stem cell research, including the use of human embryonic stem cells, is acceptable in principle in Islam because of its potential for discovering treatments for incurable diseases and injuries.
2. Because pre-implanted fertilized ova cannot develop into human beings on their own, they are not human life according to Islamic law.
3. Using excess embryos from in vitro fertilization for stem cell research is permissible. Normally, these embryos would be discarded or left to die.
4. Creating human embryos solely for research is prohibited in Islamic law.

## PRACTICAL STEPS FOR CARING FOR MUSLIM PATIENTS

Stem cells from spare embryos of fertility-clinic couples some day may yield treatments for many serious illnesses and injuries. Most Islamic scholars vigorously support embryonic stem cell research, but insist that medical science professionals conduct the research within strict religious regulations.

### Before Talking with the Patient and Her Family

1. Read the "Islamic Perspective on Stem Cell Research" section.
2. Query healthcare providers about the patient's medical and emotional states, and her husband's and family's, and about their attitudes toward stem cell research and donation.

### Once with the Patient and Her Family

1. Encourage the patient and her family to contact their imam or religious leader for support.
2. Assess the mindset of the patient and her husband about donating stem cell tissue from pre-implanted fertilized ova, afterbirth tissue, or a spontaneously aborted fetus.
3. If the stem cell tissue comes from an aborted fetus, consult the "Abortion" chapter about the care of the fetus.
4. Check in with the couple's families. They may be involved in the situation and decision.
5. Help educate the Muslim couple and families about the positive aspects of stem cell donation.
6. Support the Muslim couple in their final decision.
7. Offer prayer, if the family desires. See "Supplications (*ad'iya*)," Appendix 3. Ask the patient and family if they want a chaplain or healthcare worker to read the prayers in English or if they want to recite the Qur'an themselves. They also may want to make supplication (*du'a*) privately. If so, provide them with copies of the prayers. Some Muslims are offended if non-Muslims read the Qur'an. Never invoke the name of Jesus in prayers; this also is offensive to Muslims. Muslims pray only to God.

NOTES

[1] Abdul Sachedina, *Islamic Biomedical Ethics: Principles and Applications,* (Oxford: Oxford University Press, 2009), 214. (Note: Sachedina, while writing about the majority view, opposes it. See 212-15.)

[2] Ibid., 138.

[3] Ibid., 212.

[4] Muhammad ibn Ismail al-Bukhari, *Sahih Bukhari,* Vol. 4, Book 55, Number 549, University of Southern California *ahadith* database: http://www.usc.edu/schools/college/crcc/engagement/resources/texts/muslim/hadith/bukhari/052.sbt.html. Accessed 4 April 2010.

[5] Abdul Sachedina, 215.

[6] Ibid., 213.

[7] Abu Dawud, *Sunan Abu-Dawud,* Book 28, Number 3865, University of Southern California *ahadith* database:
http://www.usc.edu/schools/college/crcc/engagement/resources/texts/muslim/hadith/abudawuda/028.sat.html. Accessed 21 December 2009.

[8] S. Askoy, "Making regulations and drawing up legislation in Islamic countries under conditions of uncertainty, with special reference to embryonic stem cell research," *Journal of Medical Ethics* 2005; 31: 399–403. doi: 10.1136/jme.2003.005827, http://ukpmc.ac.uk/articlerender.cgi?artid=1565514. Accessed 21 December 2009.

[9] Abdul Sachedina, 214.

[10] IMANA Ethics Committee, *Stem Cell Research: The IMANA Perspective,* (Lombard, IL: Islamic Medical Association of North America, n.d.), page 11. According to this IMANA article, the same ruling mentioned above "was expressed in many resolutions, including that of the First International Conference in Bioethics in the Muslim World, Cairo, 12/10-13, 1991, the Fiqh Council of North America, International Institute of Islamic Thought, USA, Islamic Organization of Medical Sciences (IOMS), the Society of Islamic Medical Sciences of the Syndicate of Jordanian Physicians Conference of September 2000 and the Muslim World League's Islamic Fiqh Council."

[11] Ibid.

# APPENDIX 1

# PRACTICAL STEPS AT THE DEATH OF A MUSLIM PATIENT

The family members or designated spokesperson of a deceased loved one may request that the funeral home, Islamic center, or mosque complete the final arrangements. However, they may want to handle these arrangements themselves. Regardless, it is important that those preparing the body for burial are aware of the cultural or faith needs of the family. In Islam, for example, the body of the deceased must be buried immediately and must not be autopsied, embalmed, or undergo other Westernized funeral procedures. Do not cut the deceased's nails and hair, for example.

1. Healthcare workers should follow required protocol for the disposition of a body from the respective healthcare facility.
2. The pastoral care department should provide the grieving family with a list of Muslim funeral homes, local mosques, and Islamic centers that offer the washing (*ghusl*) and shrouding (*kafan*) of the dead and a list of cemeteries with Muslim burial plots. In the grave, the deceased person's head always faces Mecca, Saudi Arabia.
3. Family members or the designated spokesperson should
   – Complete and register the death certificate with local government authorities
   – Obtain a burial certificate
   – Notify the funeral home and provide the funeral home with the death certificate

– Arrange for washing (*ghusl*), shrouding in a cloth (*kafan*), and burial of the deceased person with the funeral home, local mosque, or Islamic center.

– Some hospitals permit the washing to be done at the hospital before the transport of the body. The chaplain or healthcare worker should see if this can be accommodated.

– Select a grave marker at the funeral home (a grave with a simple headstone to mark the grave, according to *shari'a*).

– Schedule *janazah* (funeral prayer) with the local mosque or Islamic center.

– Arrange transport of deceased person to janazah prayer ceremony and cemetery.

– Arrange for the burial ceremony.

## APPENDIX 2

# WELCOMING A NEW BORN BABY (*AQIQAH*)

### UPON BIRTH

1. A parent or guardian (usually a male) of the child quietly says the Islamic call to prayer (*adhan*) in the right ear of the baby. The *adhan* is: "*Allahu Akbar* (Allah is Great), repeated four times; *Ash-hadu an la ilaha illa Llah* (I bear witness that there is no god except the One God), repeated twice; *Ash-hadu anna Muhammadan rasulu Llah* (I bear witness that Muhammad is the messenger of Allah), repeated twice; *Hayya 'ala-s-salah* (Rise up for prayer), repeated twice; *Hayya 'ala-l-falah* (Rise up for Salvation), repeated twice; *Allahu Akbar* (Allah is Great), repeated twice; and *La ilaha illa Llah* (There is no god except the One God).
2. A respected elder of the family rubs a small piece of soft date gently on the baby's palette. Honey is used, if a date is unavailable.
3. Some Muslims place a small pouch containing a prayer around the baby's neck or wrist by a black string. This item is considered sacred, is for protection of the baby, and should not be removed unless medically necessary.
4. A supplication (*du'a*) for a life to be lived unto God is made for the baby.

### ON THE SEVENTH DAY

1. Family and friends gather for specially prepared foods; an animal is slaughtered ritually, cooked, and served to the poor and/or to friends and family; gifts are given to the baby and/or the baby's parents.

2. The baby is named.
3. The baby's hair is shaved and a donation of money is given to the poor. The amount of the donation is based on the silver standard and according to the weight of the baby's hair. This ritual symbolizes the innocence of the baby. If the child's skull is too soft, strongly encourage the parents to wait. Get the support of a physician, if needed.
4. A baby boy is circumcised.

## APPENDIX 3

# SUPPLICATIONS (*AD'IYA*)

Muslims love to pray. They pray in times of need, distress, personal loss and tragedy – and when thankful for the restored health of a loved one or for the birth of a baby. Prayer is an invitation to God. In Qur'an 40:60, God says: ". . . your Sustainer says: 'Call on Me, [and] I shall respond to you!'" In supplication (*du'a*) to God, Muslims recite verses (*ayat*) from Islam's holiest of books, the Qur'an, and repeat the sayings (*ahadith*) of Prophet Muhammad, adding their own words to the *du'a*. Most Muslims recite the Qur'an in Arabic, the canonical language of the holy book, while performing *du'a* and making ritual prayer (*salah*). Some do not. Along with the Arabic, English translations and transliterations, some oft-recited *ayat* and *hadith*, sg./*ahadith*, pl. are provided below. Qur'anic recitation of ayat differs culturally. Consult with the patient or family members about choosing the most appropriate scripture.

A simple transliteration system of accents, under-dots, and underscores facilitates the reading of the following Qur'anic scripture and *ahadith*. The transliteration guide is as follows: Read a<as in bat; i< as in beet; u< as in boot. Hold these letters two counts. Emphatic letters ( h{, s{, d{, t{, dh{, and q{ ) are pronounced with an echo or thud.

## Appendix 3

### *Sura Fatihah*, Qur'an 1:1-7

In the Name of God, The Most Gracious, The Dispenser of Grace

"In the name of God, The Most Gracious, the Dispenser of Grace: All praise is due to God alone, the Sustainer of all the worlds, the Most Gracious, the Dispenser of Grace, Lord of the Day of Judgment! Thee alone do we worship, and untoThee alone do we turn for aid. Guide us the straight way –the way of those upon whom Thou hast bestowed Thy blessings, not of those who have been condemned [by Thee], nor of those who go astray

Bismi'Llāhi'l-raḥmāni'l-raḥīm.

Al-ḥamdu li'l-Lāhi rabbi'l-`ālamīn. Al-raḥmāni'l-raḥīm. Māliki yawmi'l-dīn. Iyyāka na'budu wa-iyyāka nasta'īn. Ihdinā'l-ṣirāṭa'l-mustaqim. Ṣirāṭa'lladhīna an'amta 'alayhi ghayri'l-maghḍūbi 'alayhim wa-lā'l-ḍāllin.

بِسمِ ٱللهِ ٱلرَّحمَـٰنِ ٱلرَّحِيمِ

ٱلحَمدُ لِلَّهِ رَبِّ ٱلعَـٰلَمِينَ ٱلرَّحمَـٰنِ ٱلرَّحِيمِ مَـٰلِكِ يَومِ ٱلدِّينِ إِيَّاكَ نَعبُدُ وَإِيَّاكَ نَستَعِينُ ٱهدِنَا ٱلصِّرَٲطَ ٱلمُستَقِيمَ صِرَٲطَ ٱلَّذِينَ أَنعَمتَ عَلَيهِم غَيرِ ٱلمَغضُوبِ عَلَيهِم وَلَا ٱلضَّآلِّينَ

### *Sura Baqara, Qur'an* 2:153

In the Name of God, The Most Gracious, The Dispenser of Grace

"O you who have attained to faith! Seek aid in steadfast patience and prayer: for, behold, God is with those who are patient in adversity."

Bismi'Llāhi'l-raḥmāni'l-raḥīm.

Yā ayyuhā'lladhīna āmanū'sta`īnu bi'l-ṣabri wa'l-ṣalāti inna'Llāha ma`a'l-ṣābirīn

بِسمِ ٱللهِ ٱلرَّحمَـٰنِ ٱلرَّحِيمِ

يَا أَيُّهَا الَّذِينَ آمَنُواْ اسْتَعِينُواْ بِالصَّبْرِ وَالصَّلاَةِ إِنَّ اللهَ مَعَ الصَّابِرِينَ

*Sura Baqara*, Qur'an 2:186

In the Name of God, The Most Gracious, The Dispenser of Grace

"And if My servants ask thee about Me – behold, I am near; I respond to the call of him who calls, whenever he calls unto Me: let them, then, respond unto Me, and believe in Me, so that they might follow the right way."

Bismi'Llahi'l-raḥmani'l-raḥim

wa-idha sa'alaka `ibadi `anni fa-inni qaribun ujibu da`wata'l-da`i idha da`ani fal-yastajibu li wal-yu'minu bi la`allahum yarshudun

بسم الله الرحمن الرحيم

وَإِذَا سَأَلَكَ عِبَادِي عَنِّي فَإِنِّي قَرِيبٌ أُجِيبُ دَعْوَةَ الدَّاعِ إِذَا دَعَانِ فَلْيَسْتَجِيبُواْ لِي وَلْيُؤْمِنُواْ
بِي لَعَلَّهُمْ يَرْشُدُونَ

*Sura Baqara*, Qur'an 2:255

In the name of God, The Most Gracious, The Dispenser of Grace

"God - There is no deity save Him, the Ever-Living, the Self-Subsistent Fount of All Being. Neither slumber overtakes Him, nor sleep. His is all that is in the heavens and all that is on earth. Who is there could intercede with Him, unless it be by His leave? He knows all that lies open before men and all that is hidden from them, whereas they cannot attain to aught of His knowledge save that which He wills [them to attain]. His eternal power overspreads the heavens and the earth, and their upholding wearies Him not. And he alone is truly exalted, tremendous."

# Appendix 3

Bismi'l-Lāhi'l-raḥmāni'l-raḥīm

Allāhu lā ilāha illā huwa'l-ḥayyu'l-qayyūmu lā ta'khudhuhu sinatun wa-lā nawmun lahu mā fī'l-samawāti wa-mā fī'l-arḍi man dha'lladhī yashfa'u 'indahu illā bi-idhnihi ya'lamu ma bayna aydihim wa-mā khalfahum wa-lā yuḥitūna bi-shay'in min 'ilmihi illā bi-ma sha'a wasi`a kursiyyuhu'l-samāwati wa'l-arḍa wa-lā ya'uduhu ḥifẓuhumā wa-huwa'l-Aliyyu'l-'aẓim

بسم الله الرحمن الرحيم

اللَّهُ لا إِلَٰهَ إِلاَّ هُوَ الْحَيُّ الْقَيُّومُ ۚ لا تَأْخُذُهُ سِنَةٌ وَلا نَوْمٌ ۚ لَهُ مَا فِي السَّمَاوَاتِ وَمَا فِي الْأَرْضِ ۗ مَنْ ذَا الَّذِي يَشْفَعُ عِنْدَهُ إِلا بِإِذْنِهِ ۚ يَعْلَمُ مَا بَيْنَ أَيْدِيهِمْ وَمَا خَلْفَهُمْ ۖ وَلا يُحِيطُونَ بِشَيْءٍ مِنْ عِلْمِهِ إِلا بِمَا شَاءَ ۚ وَسِعَ كُرْسِيُّهُ السَّمَاوَاتِ وَالأرْضَ ۖ وَلا يَئُودُهُ حِفْظُهُمَا ۚ وَهُوَ الْعَلِيُّ الْعَظِيمُ

## *Sura Baqara,* Qur'an 2:285

In the Name of God, The Most Gracious, The Dispenser of Grace

"The Apostle, and the believers with him believe in what has been bestowed upon him from on high by his Sustainer: they all believe in God, and His angels, and His revelations, and His apostles, making no distinction between any of His apostles; and they say: 'We have heard, and we pay heed. Grant us Thy forgiveness, O our Sustainer, for with Thee is all journeys' end!' "

Bismi'l-Lāhi'l-raḥmāni'l-raḥīm

Āmana'l-rasūlu bi-mā unzila ilayhi min rabbihi wa'l-mu'minūna kullun āmana bi'Llāhi wa-mala'ikatihi wa-kutubihi wa-rusulihi lā nufarriqu bayna aḥadin min rusulihi wa-qālu sami`nā wa-aṭa`nā ghufrānaka rabbanā wa-ilayka'l-maṣir

بسم الله الرحمن الرحيم

آمَنَ الرَّسُولُ بِمَا أُنْزِلَ إِلَيْهِ مِنْ رَبِّهِ وَالْمُؤْمِنُونَ ۚ كُلٌّ آمَنَ بِاللَّهِ وَمَلائِكَتِهِ وَكُتُبِهِ وَرُسُلِهِ لا نُفَرِّقُ بَيْنَ أَحَدٍ مِنْ رُسُلِهِ ۚ وَقَالُوا سَمِعْنَا وَأَطَعْنَا ۖ غُفْرَانَكَ رَبَّنَا وَإِلَيْكَ الْمَصِيرُ

## *Sura Baqara,* Qur'an 2:286

In the Name of God, The Most Gracious, The Dispenser of Grace

"God does not burden any human being with more than he is well able to bear: in his favour shall be whatever good he does, and against him whatever evil he does. O our Sustainer! Take us not to task if we forget or unwittingly do wrong! O our Sustainer! Lay not upon us a burden such as Thou didst lay upon those who lived before us! O our Sustainer! Make us not bear burdens which we have no strength to bear! And efface Thou our sins, and grant us forgiveness, and bestow Thy mercy upon us! Thou art our Lord Supreme: succour us, then, against people who deny the truth!"

Bismi'l-Lāhi'l-raḥmāni'l-raḥīm

Lā yukallifu'Llāhu nafsan illā wus`ahā lahā mā kasabat rabbanā lā tu'ākhidhnā in nasīnā aw akhṭa'nā rabbanā wa-lā taḥmil `alaynā iṣran kamā ḥamaltahu `alā'lladhīna min qablinā rabbanā wa-lā tuḥmilnā mā lā ṭāqata la-nā bi-hi wa'fu `annā wa'ghfir la-nā wa'rḥamnā anta mawlānā fa'nṣurnā `alā'l-qawmi'l-kāfirīn

بسم الله الرحمن الرحيم

لا يُكَلِّفُ اللَّهُ نَفْسًا إِلا وُسْعَهَا ۚ لَهَا مَا كَسَبَتْ وَعَلَيْهَا مَا اكْتَسَبَتْ ۗ رَبَّنَا لا تُؤَاخِذْنَا إِنْ نَسِينَا أَوْ أَخْطَأْنَا ۚ رَبَّنَا وَلا تَحْمِلْ عَلَيْنَا إِصْرًا كَمَا حَمَلْتَهُ عَلَى الَّذِينَ مِنْ قَبْلِنَا ۚ رَبَّنَا وَلا تُحَمِّلْنَا مَا لا طَاقَةَ لَنَا بِهِ ۖ وَاعْفُ عَنَّا وَاغْفِرْ لَنَا وَارْحَمْنَا ۚ أَنْتَ مَوْلانَا فَانْصُرْنَا عَلَى الْقَوْمِ الْكَافِرِينَ

## Sura Ya-Sin, Qur'an 36: 1-83

In the Name of God, The Most Gracious, The Dispenser of Grace

36:1 O thou human being!

36:2 Consider this Qur'an full of wisdom:

36:3 verily, thou art indeed one of God's message-bearers,

36:4 pursuing a straight way

36:5 by [virtue of] what is being bestowed from on high by the Almighty, the Dispenser of Grace,

36:6 [bestowed upon thee] so that thou mayest warn people whose forefathers had not been warned, and who therefore are unaware [of the meaning of right and wrong].

36:7 Indeed, the word [of God's condemnation] is bound to come true against most of them: for they will not believe.

36:8 Behold, around their necks We have put shackles, reaching up to their chins, so that their heads are forced up;

36:9 and We have set a barrier before them and a barrier behind them, and We have enshrouded them in veils so that they cannot see:

36:10 thus, it is all one to them whether thou warnest them or dost not warn them: they will not believe.

36:11 Thou canst [truly] warn only him who is willing to take the reminder to heart, and who stands in awe of the Most Gracious although He is beyond the reach of human perception: unto such, then, give the glad tiding of [God's] forgiveness and of a most excellent reward!

36:12 Verily, We shall indeed bring the dead back to life; and We shall record whatever [deeds] they have sent ahead, and the traces [of good and evil] which they have left behind: for of all things do We take account in a record clear.

36:13 And set forth unto them a parable - [the story of how] the people of a township [behaved] when [Our] message-bearers came unto them.

36:14 Lo! We sent unto them two [apostles], and. they gave the lie to both; and so We strengthened [the two] with a third; and thereupon they said: "Behold, we have been sent unto you [by God]!"

36:15 [The others] answered: "You are nothing but mortal men like ourselves; moreover, the Most Gracious has never bestowed aught [of revelation]

from on high. You do nothing but lie!"

36:16 Said [the apostles]: "Our Sustainer knows that we have indeed been sent unto you;

36:17 but we are not bound to do more than clearly deliver the message [entrusted to us]."

36:18 Said [the others]: "Truly, we augur evil from you! Indeed, if you desist not, we will surely stone you, and grievous suffering is bound to befall you at our hands!"

36:19 [The apostles] replied: "Your destiny, good or evil, is [bound up] with yourselves! [Does it seem evil to you] if you are told to take [the truth] to heart? Nay, but you are people who have wasted their own selves!"

36:20 At that, a man came running from the farthest end of the city, [and] exclaimed: "O my people! Follow these message-bearers!

36:21 Follow those who ask no reward of you, and themselves are rightly guided!

36:22 "[As for me,] why should I not worship Him who has brought me into being, and to whom you all will be brought back?

36:23 Should I take to worshipping [other] deities beside Him? [But then,] if the Most Gracious should will that harm befall me, their intercession could not in the least avail me, nor could they save me:

36:24 and so, behold, I would have indeed, most obviously, lost myself in error!

36:25 "Verily, [O my people,] in the Sustainer of you all have I come to believe: listen, then, to me!"

36:26 [And] he was told, "[Thou shalt] enter paradise!" - [whereupon] he exclaimed: "Would that my people knew

36:27 how my Sustainer has forgiven me [the sins of my past], and has placed me among the honoured ones!"

36:28 And after that, no host out of heaven did We send down against his people, nor did We need to send down any:
36:29 nothing was [needed] but one single blast [of Our punishment] - and lo! they became as still and silent as ashes.

36:30 Oh, the regrets that [most] human beings will have to bear! Never has an apostle come to them without their deriding him!

36:31 Are they not aware of how many a generation We have destroyed before their time, [and] that those [that have perished] will never return to them,

36:32 and [that] all of them, all together, will [in the end] before Us be arraigned?

36:33 And [yet,] they have a sign [of Our power to create and to resurrect] in the lifeless earth which We make alive, and out of which We bring forth grain, whereof they may eat;

36:34 and [how] We make gardens of date-palms and vines [grow] thereon, and cause springs to gush [forth] within it,

36:35 so that they may eat of the fruit thereof, though it was not their hands that made it. Will they not, then, be grateful?

36:36 Limitless in His glory is He who has created opposites in whatever the earth produces, and in men's own selves, and in that of which [as yet] they have no knowledge.

36:37 And [of Our sway over all that exists] they have a sign in the night: We withdraw from it the [light of] day - and lo! they are in darkness.

36:38 And [they have a sign in] the sun: it runs in an orbit of its own [and] that is laid down by the will of the Almighty, the All-Knowing;

36:39 and [in] the moon, for which We have determined phases [which it must traverse] till it becomes like an old date-stalk, dried-up and curved:

36:40 [and] neither may the sun overtake the moon, nor can the night usurp the time of day, since all of them float through space [in accordance with Our laws].

36:41 And [it ought to be] a sign for them that We bear their offspring [over the seas] in laden ships,

36:42 and [that] We create for them things of a similar kind, on which they may embark [in their travels];

36:43 and [that,] if such be Our will, We may cause them to drown, with none to respond to their cry for help: and [then] they cannot be saved,

36:44 unless it be by an act of mercy from Us and a grant of life for a [further span of] time.

36:45 And [yet,] when they are told, "Beware of [God's insight into] all that lies open before you and all that is hidden from you, so that you might be graced with His mercy," [most men choose to remain deaf;]

36:46 and no message of their Sustainer's messages ever reaches them without their turning away from it.

36:47 Thus, when they are told, "Spend on others out of what God has provided for you as sustenance," those who are bent on denying the truth say unto those who believe, "Shall we feed anyone whom, if [your] God had so willed, He could have fed [Himself]? Clearly, you are but lost in error!"

36:48 And they add, "When is this promise [of resurrection] to be fulfilled? [Answer this] if you are men of truth!"

36:49 [And they are unaware that] nothing awaits them beyond a single blast [of God's punishment], which will overtake them while they are still arguing – [against resurrection]:

36:50 and so [sudden will be their end that] no testament will they be able to make, – nor to their own people will they return!

36:51 And [then] the trumpet [of resurrection] will be blown – and lo! out of their graves towards their Sustainer will they all rush forth!

36:52 They will say: "Oh, woe unto us! Who has roused us from our sleep [of death]?" [Whereupon they will be told:] "This is what the Most Gracious has promised! And His message-bearers spoke the truth!"

36:53 Nothing will there have been but one single blast and lo! before Us will all of them be arraigned [and be told]:

36:54 "Today, then, no human being shall be wronged in the least, nor shalt you be requited for aught but what you were doing [on earth].

36:55 "Behold, those who are destined for paradise shall today have joy in whatever they do:

36:56 in happiness will they and their spouses on couches recline;

36:57 [only] delight will there be for them, and theirs shall be all that they could ask for:

36:58 peace and fulfillment through the word of a Sustainer who dispenses all grace.

36:59 "But stand aside today, O you who were lost in sin!

36:60 Did I not enjoin on you, O you children of Adam, that you should not worship Satan – since, verily, he is your open foe

36:61 and that you should worship Me [alone]? This would have been a straight way!

36:62 And [as for Satan] he had already led astray a great many of you: could you not, then, use your reason?

36:63 "This, then, is the hell of which you were warned again and again:

36:64 endure it today as an outcome of your persistent denial of the truth!"

36:65 On that Day We shall set a seal on their mouths but their hands will speak unto Us, and their feet will bear witness to whatever they have earned [in life].

36:66 Now had it been on Our will [that men should not be able to discern between right and wrong], We could surely have deprived them of their sight, so that they would stray forever from the [right] way: for how could they have had insight [into what is true]?

36:67 And had it been Our will [that they should not be free to choose between right and wrong], We could surely have given them a different nature [and created them as beings rooted] in their places, so that they would not be able to move forward, and could not turn back.

36:68 But [let them always remember that] if We lengthen a human being's days, We also cause him to decline in his powers [when he grows old]: will they not, then, use their reason?

36:69 And [thus it is:] We have not imparted to this [Prophet the gift of] poetry, nor would [poetry] have suited this [message]: it is but a reminder and a [divine] discourse, clear in itself and clearly showing the truth,

36:70 to the end that it may warn everyone who is alive [of heart], and that the word [of God] may bear witness against all who deny the truth.

36:71 Are they, then, not aware that it is for them that We have created, among all the things which Our hands have wrought, the domestic animals of which they are [now] masters?

36:72 and that We have subjected them to men's will, so that some of them they may use for riding and of some they may eat,

36:73 and may have [yet other] benefits from them, and [milk] to drink? Will they not, then, be grateful?

36:74 But [nay,] they take to worshipping deities other than God, [hoping] to be succoured [by them, and not knowing that]

36:75 they are unable to succour their devotees, even though to them they may [appear to] be hosts drawn up [for succour].

36:76 However, be not grieved by the sayings of those [who deny the truth]: verily, We know all that they keep secret as well as all that they bring into the open.

36:77 Is man, then, not aware that it is We who create him out of a [mere] drop of sperm – whereupon, lo! he shows himself endowed with the power to think and to argue?

36:78 And [now] he [argues about Us, and] thinks of Us in terms of comparison, and is oblivious of how he himself was created! [And so] he says, "Who could give life to bones that have crumbled to dust?"

36:79 Say: "He who brought them into being in the first instance will give them life [once again], seeing that He has full knowledge of every act of creation:

36:80 He who produces for you fire out of the green tree, so that, lo! you kindle [your fires] therewith."

36:81 Is, then, He who has created the heavens and the earth not able to create [anew] the like of those [who have died]? Yea, indeed – for He alone is the all-knowing Creator:

36:82 His Being alone is such that when He wills a thing to be, He but says unto it, "Be"–and it is.

36:83 Limitless, then, in His glory is He in whose hand rests the mighty dominion over all things; and unto Him you all will be brought back!

## سُورَةُ يسٓ

بِسْمِ ٱللَّهِ ٱلرَّحْمَٰنِ ٱلرَّحِيمِ

يسٓ (١) وَٱلْقُرْءَانِ ٱلْحَكِيمِ (٢) إِنَّكَ لَمِنَ ٱلْمُرْسَلِينَ (٣) عَلَىٰ صِرَٰطٍ مُّسْتَقِيمٍ
(٤) تَنزِيلَ ٱلْعَزِيزِ ٱلرَّحِيمِ (٥) لِتُنذِرَ قَوْمًا مَّآ أُنذِرَ ءَابَآؤُهُمْ فَهُمْ غَٰفِلُونَ (٦)
لَقَدْ حَقَّ ٱلْقَوْلُ عَلَىٰٓ أَكْثَرِهِمْ فَهُمْ لَا يُؤْمِنُونَ (٧) إِنَّا جَعَلْنَا فِىٓ أَعْنَٰقِهِمْ أَغْلَٰلًا
فَهِىَ إِلَى ٱلْأَذْقَانِ فَهُم مُّقْمَحُونَ (٨) وَجَعَلْنَا مِنۢ بَيْنِ أَيْدِيهِمْ سَدًّا وَمِنْ خَلْفِهِمْ
سَدًّا فَأَغْشَيْنَٰهُمْ فَهُمْ لَا يُبْصِرُونَ (٩) وَسَوَآءٌ عَلَيْهِمْ ءَأَنذَرْتَهُمْ أَمْ لَمْ تُنذِرْهُمْ لَا
يُؤْمِنُونَ (١٠) إِنَّمَا تُنذِرُ مَنِ ٱتَّبَعَ ٱلذِّكْرَ وَخَشِىَ ٱلرَّحْمَٰنَ بِٱلْغَيْبِ فَبَشِّرْهُ
بِمَغْفِرَةٍ وَأَجْرٍ كَرِيمٍ (١١) إِنَّا نَحْنُ نُحْىِ ٱلْمَوْتَىٰ وَنَكْتُبُ مَا قَدَّمُوا۟
وَءَاثَٰرَهُمْ وَكُلَّ شَىْءٍ أَحْصَيْنَٰهُ فِىٓ إِمَامٍ مُّبِينٍ (١٢) وَٱضْرِبْ لَهُم مَّثَلًا
أَصْحَٰبَ ٱلْقَرْيَةِ إِذْ جَآءَهَا ٱلْمُرْسَلُونَ (١٣) إِذْ أَرْسَلْنَآ إِلَيْهِمُ ٱثْنَيْنِ فَكَذَّبُوهُمَا
فَعَزَّزْنَا بِثَالِثٍ فَقَالُوٓا۟ إِنَّآ إِلَيْكُم مُّرْسَلُونَ (١٤) قَالُوا۟ مَآ أَنتُمْ إِلَّا بَشَرٌ مِّثْلُنَا وَمَآ
أَنزَلَ ٱلرَّحْمَٰنُ مِن شَىْءٍ إِنْ أَنتُمْ إِلَّا تَكْذِبُونَ (١٥) قَالُوا۟ رَبُّنَا يَعْلَمُ إِنَّآ إِلَيْكُمْ
لَمُرْسَلُونَ (١٦) وَمَا عَلَيْنَآ إِلَّا ٱلْبَلَٰغُ ٱلْمُبِينُ (١٧) قَالُوٓا۟ إِنَّا تَطَيَّرْنَا بِكُمْ لَئِن لَّمْ
تَنتَهُوا۟ لَنَرْجُمَنَّكُمْ وَلَيَمَسَّنَّكُم مِّنَّا عَذَابٌ أَلِيمٌ (١٨) قَالُوا۟ طَٰٓئِرُكُم مَّعَكُمْ أَئِن
ذُكِّرْتُم بَلْ أَنتُمْ قَوْمٌ مُّسْرِفُونَ (١٩) وَجَآءَ مِنْ أَقْصَا ٱلْمَدِينَةِ رَجُلٌ يَسْعَىٰ قَالَ
يَٰقَوْمِ ٱتَّبِعُوا۟ ٱلْمُرْسَلِينَ (٢٠) ٱتَّبِعُوا۟ مَن لَّا يَسْـَٔلُكُمْ أَجْرًا وَهُم مُّهْتَدُونَ (٢١)
وَمَا لِىَ لَآ أَعْبُدُ ٱلَّذِى فَطَرَنِى وَإِلَيْهِ تُرْجَعُونَ (٢٢) ءَأَتَّخِذُ مِن دُونِهِۦٓ ءَالِهَةً
إِن يُرِدْنِ ٱلرَّحْمَٰنُ بِضُرٍّ لَّا تُغْنِ عَنِّى شَفَٰعَتُهُمْ شَيْـًٔا وَلَا يُنقِذُونِ (٢٣) إِنِّىٓ إِذًا
لَّفِى ضَلَٰلٍ مُّبِينٍ (٢٤) إِنِّىٓ ءَامَنتُ بِرَبِّكُمْ فَٱسْمَعُونِ (٢٥) قِيلَ ٱدْخُلِ ٱلْجَنَّةَ
قَالَ يَٰلَيْتَ قَوْمِى يَعْلَمُونَ (٢٦) بِمَا غَفَرَ لِى رَبِّى وَجَعَلَنِى مِنَ ٱلْمُكْرَمِينَ
(٢٧) ۞ وَمَآ أَنزَلْنَا عَلَىٰ قَوْمِهِۦ مِنۢ بَعْدِهِۦ مِن جُندٍ مِّنَ ٱلسَّمَآءِ وَمَا كُنَّا
مُنزِلِينَ (٢٨) إِن كَانَتْ إِلَّا صَيْحَةً وَٰحِدَةً فَإِذَا هُمْ خَٰمِدُونَ (٢٩) يَٰحَسْرَةً
عَلَى ٱلْعِبَادِ مَا يَأْتِيهِم مِّن رَّسُولٍ إِلَّا كَانُوا۟ بِهِۦ يَسْتَهْزِءُونَ (٣٠) أَلَمْ يَرَوْا۟ كَمْ
أَهْلَكْنَا قَبْلَهُم مِّنَ ٱلْقُرُونِ أَنَّهُمْ إِلَيْهِمْ لَا يَرْجِعُونَ (٣١) وَإِن كُلٌّ لَّمَّا جَمِيعٌ لَّدَيْنَا
مُحْضَرُونَ (٣٢) وَءَايَةٌ لَّهُمُ ٱلْأَرْضُ ٱلْمَيْتَةُ أَحْيَيْنَٰهَا وَأَخْرَجْنَا مِنْهَا حَبًّا فَمِنْهُ
يَأْكُلُونَ (٣٣) وَجَعَلْنَا فِيهَا جَنَّٰتٍ مِّن نَّخِيلٍ وَأَعْنَٰبٍ وَفَجَّرْنَا فِيهَا مِنَ ٱلْعُيُونِ

(٣٤) لِيَأْكُلُوا۟ مِن ثَمَرِهِۦ وَمَا عَمِلَتْهُ أَيْدِيهِمْ ۖ أَفَلَا يَشْكُرُونَ (٣٥) سُبْحَٰنَ
ٱلَّذِى خَلَقَ ٱلْأَزْوَٰجَ كُلَّهَا مِمَّا تُنۢبِتُ ٱلْأَرْضُ وَمِنْ أَنفُسِهِمْ وَمِمَّا لَا يَعْلَمُونَ
(٣٦) وَءَايَةٌ لَّهُمُ ٱلَّيْلُ نَسْلَخُ مِنْهُ ٱلنَّهَارَ فَإِذَا هُم مُّظْلِمُونَ (٣٧) وَٱلشَّمْسُ
تَجْرِى لِمُسْتَقَرٍّ لَّهَا ۚ ذَٰلِكَ تَقْدِيرُ ٱلْعَزِيزِ ٱلْعَلِيمِ (٣٨) وَٱلْقَمَرَ قَدَّرْنَٰهُ مَنَازِلَ حَتَّىٰ
عَادَ كَٱلْعُرْجُونِ ٱلْقَدِيمِ (٣٩) لَا ٱلشَّمْسُ يَنۢبَغِى لَهَآ أَن تُدْرِكَ ٱلْقَمَرَ وَلَا ٱلَّيْلُ
سَابِقُ ٱلنَّهَارِ ۚ وَكُلٌّ فِى فَلَكٍ يَسْبَحُونَ (٤٠) وَءَايَةٌ لَّهُمْ أَنَّا حَمَلْنَا ذُرِّيَّتَهُمْ فِى
ٱلْفُلْكِ ٱلْمَشْحُونِ (٤١) وَخَلَقْنَا لَهُم مِّن مِّثْلِهِۦ مَا يَرْكَبُونَ (٤٢) وَإِن نَّشَأْ
نُغْرِقْهُمْ فَلَا صَرِيخَ لَهُمْ وَلَا هُمْ يُنقَذُونَ (٤٣) إِلَّا رَحْمَةً مِّنَّا وَمَتَٰعًا إِلَىٰ حِينٍ
(٤٤) وَإِذَا قِيلَ لَهُمُ ٱتَّقُوا۟ مَا بَيْنَ أَيْدِيكُمْ وَمَا خَلْفَكُمْ لَعَلَّكُمْ تُرْحَمُونَ (٤٥) وَمَا
تَأْتِيهِم مِّنْ ءَايَةٍ مِّنْ ءَايَٰتِ رَبِّهِمْ إِلَّا كَانُوا۟ عَنْهَا مُعْرِضِينَ (٤٦) وَإِذَا قِيلَ لَهُمْ
أَنفِقُوا۟ مِمَّا رَزَقَكُمُ ٱللَّهُ قَالَ ٱلَّذِينَ كَفَرُوا۟ لِلَّذِينَ ءَامَنُوٓا۟ أَنُطْعِمُ مَن لَّوْ يَشَآءُ ٱللَّهُ
أَطْعَمَهُۥٓ إِنْ أَنتُمْ إِلَّا فِى ضَلَٰلٍ مُّبِينٍ (٤٧) وَيَقُولُونَ مَتَىٰ هَٰذَا ٱلْوَعْدُ إِن كُنتُمْ
صَٰدِقِينَ (٤٨) مَا يَنظُرُونَ إِلَّا صَيْحَةً وَٰحِدَةً تَأْخُذُهُمْ وَهُمْ يَخِصِّمُونَ (٤٩)
فَلَا يَسْتَطِيعُونَ تَوْصِيَةً وَلَآ إِلَىٰٓ أَهْلِهِمْ يَرْجِعُونَ (٥٠) وَنُفِخَ فِى ٱلصُّورِ فَإِذَا
هُم مِّنَ ٱلْأَجْدَاثِ إِلَىٰ رَبِّهِمْ يَنسِلُونَ (٥١) قَالُوا۟ يَٰوَيْلَنَا مَنۢ بَعَثَنَا مِن مَّرْقَدِنَا ۜ
هَٰذَا مَا وَعَدَ ٱلرَّحْمَٰنُ وَصَدَقَ ٱلْمُرْسَلُونَ (٥٢) إِن كَانَتْ إِلَّا صَيْحَةً وَٰحِدَةً
فَإِذَا هُمْ جَمِيعٌ لَّدَيْنَا مُحْضَرُونَ (٥٣) فَٱلْيَوْمَ لَا تُظْلَمُ نَفْسٌ شَيْـًٔا وَلَا تُجْزَوْنَ إِلَّا
مَا كُنتُمْ تَعْمَلُونَ (٥٤) إِنَّ أَصْحَٰبَ ٱلْجَنَّةِ ٱلْيَوْمَ فِى شُغُلٍ فَٰكِهُونَ (٥٥) هُمْ
وَأَزْوَٰجُهُمْ فِى ظِلَٰلٍ عَلَى ٱلْأَرَآئِكِ مُتَّكِـُٔونَ (٥٦) لَهُمْ فِيهَا فَٰكِهَةٌ وَلَهُم مَّا
يَدَّعُونَ (٥٧) سَلَٰمٌ قَوْلًا مِّن رَّبٍّ رَّحِيمٍ (٥٨) وَٱمْتَٰزُوا۟ ٱلْيَوْمَ أَيُّهَا ٱلْمُجْرِمُونَ
(٥٩) ۞ أَلَمْ أَعْهَدْ إِلَيْكُمْ يَٰبَنِىٓ ءَادَمَ أَن لَّا تَعْبُدُوا۟ ٱلشَّيْطَٰنَ ۖ إِنَّهُۥ لَكُمْ عَدُوٌّ
مُّبِينٌ (٦٠) وَأَنِ ٱعْبُدُونِى ۚ هَٰذَا صِرَٰطٌ مُّسْتَقِيمٌ (٦١) وَلَقَدْ أَضَلَّ مِنكُمْ جِبِلًّا
كَثِيرًا ۖ أَفَلَمْ تَكُونُوا۟ تَعْقِلُونَ (٦٢) هَٰذِهِۦ جَهَنَّمُ ٱلَّتِى كُنتُمْ تُوعَدُونَ (٦٣)
ٱصْلَوْهَا ٱلْيَوْمَ بِمَا كُنتُمْ تَكْفُرُونَ (٦٤) ٱلْيَوْمَ نَخْتِمُ عَلَىٰٓ أَفْوَٰهِهِمْ وَتُكَلِّمُنَآ أَيْدِيهِمْ
وَتَشْهَدُ أَرْجُلُهُم بِمَا كَانُوا۟ يَكْسِبُونَ (٦٥) وَلَوْ نَشَآءُ لَطَمَسْنَا عَلَىٰٓ أَعْيُنِهِمْ
فَٱسْتَبَقُوا۟ ٱلصِّرَٰطَ فَأَنَّىٰ يُبْصِرُونَ (٦٦) وَلَوْ نَشَآءُ لَمَسَخْنَٰهُمْ عَلَىٰ مَكَانَتِهِمْ
فَمَا ٱسْتَطَٰعُوا۟ مُضِيًّا وَلَا يَرْجِعُونَ (٦٧) وَمَن نُّعَمِّرْهُ نُنَكِّسْهُ فِى ٱلْخَلْقِ ۖ أَفَلَا
يَعْقِلُونَ (٦٨) وَمَا عَلَّمْنَٰهُ ٱلشِّعْرَ وَمَا يَنۢبَغِى لَهُۥٓ ۚ إِنْ هُوَ إِلَّا ذِكْرٌ وَقُرْءَانٌ مُّبِينٌ

(٦٩) لِّيُنذِرَ مَن كَانَ حَيًّا وَيَحِقَّ ٱلْقَوْلُ عَلَى ٱلْكَٰفِرِينَ (٧٠) أَوَلَمْ يَرَوْا۟ أَنَّا
خَلَقْنَا لَهُم مِّمَّا عَمِلَتْ أَيْدِينَآ أَنْعَٰمًا فَهُمْ لَهَا مَٰلِكُونَ (٧١) وَذَلَّلْنَٰهَا لَهُمْ فَمِنْهَا
رَكُوبُهُمْ وَمِنْهَا يَأْكُلُونَ (٧٢) وَلَهُمْ فِيهَا مَنَٰفِعُ وَمَشَارِبُ ۖ أَفَلَا يَشْكُرُونَ (٧٣)
وَٱتَّخَذُوا۟ مِن دُونِ ٱللَّهِ ءَالِهَةً لَّعَلَّهُمْ يُنصَرُونَ (٧٤) لَا يَسْتَطِيعُونَ نَصْرَهُمْ
وَهُمْ لَهُمْ جُندٌ مُّحْضَرُونَ (٧٥) فَلَا يَحْزُنكَ قَوْلُهُمْ ۘ إِنَّا نَعْلَمُ مَا يُسِرُّونَ وَمَا
يُعْلِنُونَ (٧٦) أَوَلَمْ يَرَ ٱلْإِنسَٰنُ أَنَّا خَلَقْنَٰهُ مِن نُّطْفَةٍ فَإِذَا هُوَ خَصِيمٌ مُّبِينٌ
(٧٧) وَضَرَبَ لَنَا مَثَلًا وَنَسِىَ خَلْقَهُۥ ۖ قَالَ مَن يُحْىِ ٱلْعِظَٰمَ وَهِىَ رَمِيمٌ (٧٨)
قُلْ يُحْيِيهَا ٱلَّذِىٓ أَنشَأَهَآ أَوَّلَ مَرَّةٍ ۖ وَهُوَ بِكُلِّ خَلْقٍ عَلِيمٌ (٧٩) ٱلَّذِى جَعَلَ لَكُم
مِّنَ ٱلشَّجَرِ ٱلْأَخْضَرِ نَارًا فَإِذَآ أَنتُم مِّنْهُ تُوقِدُونَ (٨٠) أَوَلَيْسَ ٱلَّذِى خَلَقَ
ٱلسَّمَٰوَٰتِ وَٱلْأَرْضَ بِقَٰدِرٍ عَلَىٰٓ أَن يَخْلُقَ مِثْلَهُم ۚ بَلَىٰ وَهُوَ ٱلْخَلَّٰقُ ٱلْعَلِيمُ (٨١)
إِنَّمَآ أَمْرُهُۥٓ إِذَآ أَرَادَ شَيْـًٔا أَن يَقُولَ لَهُۥ كُن فَيَكُونُ (٨٢) فَسُبْحَٰنَ ٱلَّذِى بِيَدِهِۦ
مَلَكُوتُ كُلِّ شَىْءٍ وَإِلَيْهِ تُرْجَعُونَ (٨٣)

## Reports of the Words of Prophet Muhammad (*ahadith*)[1]

In the Name of God, The Most Gracious, The Dispenser of Grace

"Narrated Shaddad bin Aus: The Prophet said 'The most superior way of asking for forgiveness from Allah is: *Allahumma anta Rabbi, la ilaha illa Anta, Khalaqtani wa ana 'abduka, wa ana 'ala ahdika wa wa'dika mastata'tu. Abu'u laka bini'matika, wa abu'u laka bidhanbi faghfirli, fainnahu la yaghfirudh-dhunuba illa anta. A'udhu bika min sharri ma sana'tu* [O Allah, You are my Lord; there is no God (none has the right) to be worshipped except You. You created me, and I am Your servant, and I abide to Your covenant and promise as best I can, I take refuge in You from the evil of which I have committed. I acknowledge Your favor upon me, and I acknowledge my sin, so forgive me, for verily none forgives sins except You]. If somebody recites this invocation during the night, and if he should die then, he will enter Paradise (or he will be from the people of Paradise), and if he recites it in the morning, and if he should die on the same day, he will have the same fate (i.e., will enter Paradise)."[2]

Bismi'l-Lahi'l-raḥmāni'l-raḥīm

ḥaddathanā musaddadun ḥaddathanā yazīdu ibnizuray 'ḥaddathanā ḥusaynun ḥaddathanā 'abdu'l-Lāhi ibni burayda'an bushayr ibni ka'bin 'an shaddādi ibni awsin

'an al-nabiyyi ṣallā'Llāhu 'alayhi wa-sallama qāla sayyidu'l-istighfāri'l-Lahumma anta rabbi lā ilāha illā anta khalaqtanī wa-anā 'abduka wa-anā 'alā 'ahdika wa-wa'dika mā'staṭa'tu abū'u la-ka bi-ni'matika 'alayya wa-abū'u la-ka bi-dhanbī fa'ghfir lī fa-innahu lā yaghfiru'l-dhunūbi illā anta a'udhu bi-ka min sharri mā ṣana'tu idhā qāla ḥīna yumsī fa-māta dakhala'l-jannata aw kāna min ahli'l-jannati wa-idhā qāla ḥīna yuṣbiḥu fa-mata min yawmihi mithlah

بسم الله الرحمن الرحيم

حَدَّثَنَا مُسَدَّدٌ حَدَّثَنَا يَزِيدُ بْنُ زُرَيْعٍ حَدَّثَنَا حُسَيْنٌ حَدَّثَنَا عَبْدُ اللَّهِ بْنُ بُرَيْدَةَ عَنْ بُشَيْرِ بْنِ كَعْبٍ عَنْ شَدَّادِ بْنِ أَوْسٍ

عَنْ النَّبِيِّ صَلَّى اللَّهُ عَلَيْهِ وَسَلَّمَ قَالَ سَيِّدُ الِاسْتِغْفَارِ اللَّهُمَّ أَنْتَ رَبِّي لَا إِلَهَ إِلَّا أَنْتَ خَلَقْتَنِي وَأَنَا عَبْدُكَ وَأَنَا عَلَى عَهْدِكَ وَوَعْدِكَ مَا اسْتَطَعْتُ أَبُوءُ لَكَ بِنِعْمَتِكَ عَلَيَّ وَأَبُوءُ لَكَ بِذَنْبِي فَاغْفِرْ لِي فَإِنَّهُ لَا يَغْفِرُ الذُّنُوبَ إِلَّا أَنْتَ أَعُوذُ بِكَ مِنْ شَرِّ مَا صَنَعْتُ إِذَا قَالَ حِينَ يُمْسِي فَمَاتَ دَخَلَ الْجَنَّةَ أَوْ كَانَ مِنْ أَهْلِ الْجَنَّةِ وَإِذَا قَالَ حِينَ يُصْبِحُ فَمَاتَ مِنْ يَوْمِهِ مِثْلَهُ

In the Name of God, The Most Gracious, The Dispenser of Grace

"Narrated Abu Huraira: Allah's Messenger said, 'Whoever says: '*La ilaha illallahu wahdahu la sharika lahu, lahul-mulku wa lahul-hamdu wa Huwa 'ala kulli shai'in Qadir* [There is no God (none has the right to be worshipped) except Allah, the unique, one and only with no partners. To Him belongs Dominion, and all praise is due to Him, and He has power over all things]' one hundred times will get the same reward as given for manumitting ten slaves, and one hundred good deeds will be written in his accounts, and one hundred sins will be deducted from his accounts, and it (his saying) will be a shield for him from Satan on that day till night, and nobody will be able to do a better deed except the one who does more than he." [3]

Bismi'l-Lāhi'l-raḥmāni'l-raḥīm

ḥaddathana 'abdu'l-Lāhi ibn maslamatan 'an mālikin 'an sumayyin 'an abī ṣāliḥi 'an abī hurayrata raḍiya'l-Lāhu 'anh

innā rasūla'l-Lāhi ṣallā'l-Lāhu 'alayhi wa-sallama qāla man qāla subḥāna'l-Lāhi wa-bi-ḥamdihi fī yawmin mi'atan marratin ḥuṭṭat khaṭayahu wa-in kānat mithla zabadi'l-baḥr

بسم الله الرحمن الرحيم

حَدَّثَنَا عَبْدُ اللَّهِ بْنُ مَسْلَمَةَ عَنْ مَالِكٍ عَنْ سُمَيٍّ عَنْ أَبِي صَالِحٍ عَنْ أَبِي هُرَيْرَةَ رَضِيَ اللَّهُ عَنْهُ

أَنَّ رَسُولَ اللَّهِ صَلَّى اللَّهُ عَلَيْهِ وَسَلَّمَ قَالَ مَنْ قَالَ سُبْحَانَ اللَّهِ وَبِحَمْدِهِ فِي يَوْمٍ مِائَةَ مَرَّةٍ حُطَّتْ خَطَايَاهُ وَإِنْ كَانَتْ مِثْلَ زَبَدِ الْبَحْرِ

# Appendix 3

In the Name of God, The Most Gracious, The Dispenser of Grace

"Narrated Abu Huraira: Allah's Messenger said, 'Whoever says, Subhan Allahi wa bihamdihi [Glory and praise be to Allah simultaneously] one hundred times a day, will be forgiven all his sins even if they were as much as the foam of the sea." [4]

Bismi'l-Lāhi'l-raḥmāni'l-raḥīm

ḥaddathana 'abdu'l-Lāhi ibn maslamatan 'an mālikin 'an sumayyin 'an abī ṣāliḥi 'an abī hurayrata raḍiya'l-Lāhu 'anh

innā rasūla'l-Lāhi ṣallā'l-Lāhu 'alayhi wa-sallama qāla man qāla subḥāna'l-Lāhi wa-bi-ḥamdihi fī yawmin mi'atan marratin ḥuṭṭat khaṭāyahu wa-in kānat mithla zabadi'l-baḥr

بسم الله الرحمن الرحيم

حَدَّثَنَا عَبْدُ اللَّهِ بْنُ مَسْلَمَةَ عَنْ مَالِكٍ عَنْ سُمَيٍّ عَنْ أَبِي صَالِحٍ عَنْ أَبِي هُرَيْرَةَ رَضِيَ اللَّهُ عَنْهُ

أَنَّ رَسُولَ اللَّهِ صَلَّى اللَّهُ عَلَيْهِ وَسَلَّمَ قَالَ مَنْ قَالَ سُبْحَانَ اللَّهِ وَبِحَمْدِهِ فِي يَوْمٍ مِائَةَ مَرَّةٍ حُطَّتْ خَطَايَاهُ وَإِنْ

---

NOTES

[1] The *ahadith* were selected by Aminah Assilmi on March 3, 2010. Aminah Assilmi (b. 1945 / d. 2010) was a broadcast journalist and former director of the International Union of Muslim Women.

[2] Muhammad ibn Ismail al-Bukhari, *Sahih Bukhari*, Volume 8, Book 75, Number 318, University of Southern California *ahadith* database: http://www.usc.edu/schools/college/crcc/engagement/resources/texts/muslim/hadith/bukhari/075.sbt.html>. Accessed 14 March 2010.

[3] Muhammad ibn Ismail al-Bukhari, *Sahih Bukhari*, Volume 8, Book 75, Number 412, from the University of Southern California *ahadith* database: http://www.usc.edu/schools/college/crcc/engagement/resources/texts/muslim/hadith/bukhari/075.sbt.html>. Accessed 14 March 2010.

[4] Muhammad ibn Ismail al-Bukhari, *Sahih Bukhari*, Volume 8, Book 75, Number 414, from the University of Southern California *ahadith* database, http://www.usc.edu/schools/college/crcc/engagement/resources/texts/muslim/hadith/bukhari/075.sbt.html>. Accessed 14 March 2010.

## APPENDIX 4

# COMMONLY USED EXPRESSIONS

Muslims are ever mindful of their need for God. They keep the name of God on their tongues and hearts throughout their day. A simple transliteration system of accents and under-dots facilitates the pronunciation of commonly used expressions.

The transliteration guide is as follows: Read a, ā as in bat; i, ī, as in beet; u, ū, as in boot. Hold these letters two counts. Emphatic letters (ḥ, ṣ, ḍ, ṭ, dḥ, and q) are pronounced with an echo or thud.

1. Greeting others with *assalāmu 'alaykum* (peace be unto you); the response to this greeting is *wa 'alaykum assalām* (and peace be unto you)
2. Saying *Bismillāh Ar-Raḥmān Ar-Raḥīm* (in the name of God, the Singularly Most Compassionate and Most Merciful) before meals and before undertaking any endeavor
3. Thanking God *(Ḥamdulillāh)* for difficulty and ease
4. Qualifying intended human actions or wishes for good health, a good marriage, for example, by saying *Inshā'Allāh* (if God wills)
5. Praising God *(Subḥānallāh)*
6. Expressing happiness or amazement *(Māshallāh)* upon hearing good news
7. Affirming there is no god but God *(Lā ilāha illā Llāh)*
8. Affirming Prophet Muhammad is the messenger of God *(Muḥammadun Rasūlu Llāh)*
9. Saying there is none greater than God *(Allāhu Akbar)*

10. Asking God for forgiveness *(Astaghfiru Llāh)* for a wrong or an offense committed
11. Acknowledging that only God knows *(Allāhu A'lam)* what is going to happen
12. Asking God to reward someone for a good deed done for you *(jazaka Llāhu khairan)*
13. Beseeching God for help in times of distress or need *(Yā Allāh!)*
14. Paying respect to the prophets after saying their names *(sallā Llāhu 'alayhi wa salām)*, as encouraged by Qur'an 33:56 and *aḥādīth* (reports of the words and actions of Prophet Muhammad)

APPENDIX 5

# ON LINE RESOURCES (AS OF MAY 2011)

## ABOUT ISLAMIC CHAPLAINCY

### Muslim Chaplains Association

http://muslimchaplains.org/

Provides support for Muslim chaplains working at schools, prisons, hospitals, and in the military, and for chaplains of all faiths working with Muslims

Hartford Seminary Islamic Chaplaincy Program

http://macdonald.hartsem.edu/chaplaincy/index.htm

Is the only accredited Islamic chaplaincy program in North America; offers articles and other resources

### About Islam and Muslims

IslamiCity

http://www.islamicity.com/

Provides a comprehensive overview of Islam and Muslims, and offers audio, Arabic, and English translations of Qur'an

Islamic Finder
http://www.islamicfinder.org/
Provides worldwide prayer times and information about mosques, Islamic organizations and centers, and Muslim-owned businesses

Islam for Today
http://www.islamfortoday.com/
Offers a plethora of information about the religion of Islam, Muslim history and civilizations, the rights of women in Islam, and Islam in the West

### About Islam and Medicine

Islam-USA
http://www.islam-usa.com/index.php?option=com_content&view=category&id=68&Itemid=137
Provides healthcare-related online books and articles by Shahid Attar, M.D., a member of the Islamic Society of North America, and a leading spokesperson on healthcare issues from an Islamic perspective

Islamic Medical Association of North America (IMANA)
http://www.imana.org/education.html
Provides educational materials about Islamic medical ethics

Islamic Medicine
http://www.islamicmedicine.org/
Covers a broad range of Islamic medical topics

Islamic Organization for Medical Sciences [IOMS]
http://www.islamset.com/ioms/main.html
Owns library medical articles on an array of subjects

American Muslim Health Professionals (AMHP)
http://www.amhp.us
Provides resources for improving public health, through efforts inspired by Islamic tradition

Islamic Philosophy
http://www.muslimphilosophy.com/
Houses hundreds of full-length books and articles on Islamic philosophy

Religious Opinions (*fatwas*)
http://www.islamonline.net/en/Page/Home/
Provides online library of religious opinions from Islamic jurists, and a forum for querying Muslim scholars about particular issues

**About U.S. Muslim Organizations**

Council on American Islamic Relations (CAIR)
453 New Jersey Avenue, S.E.
Washington, DC 20003
Tel: 202-488-8787
Fax: 202-488-0833
www.cair.com

Islamic Medical Association of North America (IMANA)
101 W. 22nd St., Suite 106
Lombard, IL 60148
Tel: 630-932-0000
Fax: 630-932-0005
www.imana.org

Islamic Society of North America (ISNA)
P.O. Box 38
Plainfield, IN 46168
Tel: 317-839-8157
Fax: 317-839-1840
www.isna.net

## APPENDIX 6

# GLOSSARY

**adhan**: the call to five-times daily prayer (salah)

**ajal**: the appointed death of a person

**'Ali ibn Abu Talib**: the cousin and son-in-law of Prophet Muhammad

**al-akhira:** the Hereafter or Afterlife

**Allah:** the One God, the Supreme Being

**aqiqah:** a recommended (sunna) or welcoming consecration ceremony for a newborn baby

**'azl:** coitus interruptus

**bala**: a trial or test from God

**burqa:** full-body garb worn by some Muslim women

**caliph:** successor to Prophet Muhammad, political leader of the early Muslim community

**Companions:** the followers of Prophet Muhammad; some of them accompanied him on the migration from Mecca to Yathrib (Medina) in 622 C.E.

**dhikr:** a spiritual practice of remembering the name of Allah

**du'a** (sg.), **ad'iya** (pl.): personal, informal prayer

**'Id al-Adha:** Feast of Sacrifice celebrated towards the end of the annual pilgrimage to Mecca (hajj), and commemorates the willingness of Prophet Abraham to sacrifice his son Isma'il in obedience to God

**'Id al-Fitr:** Three-day festival at the end of fasting during the month of Ramadan

**fard:** anything deemed obligatory upon Muslims by Islamic law, such as fasting during the month of Ramadan or the five daily prayers

**fard al-kifaya:** obligatory responsibilities for the entire Muslim community

**fatwa:** a religious opinion of an Islamic jurist

**fitnah:** trials or temptations

**fitra:** the innate state of purity and goodness with which humans are born

**fuqaha:** Islamic jurists

**ghusl:** a ritual purity practice of allowing clean running water to course over the entire body

**hadith** (sg.)/**ahadith** (pl.): reports of the words and actions of Prophet Muhammad and his followers (who also were called Companions); the ahadith inform us about the Sunna (the way) of Prophet Muhammad

**hajj:** annual pilgrimage of Muslims to Mecca that takes place during the eighth through thirteenth days of the last month of the Islamic year

**halal:** anything permitted by the Qur'an, the Sunna (actions and words of Prophet Muhammad), or the religious legal opinions of Islamic jurists, such as eating herbivore animals slaughtered according to Islamic guidelines

**Hanafi:** one of the four major schools of religious jurisprudence/thought in Islam; the other three are Hanbali, Maliki, and Shafi'i schools

**Hanbali:** one of the four major schools of religious jurisprudence /thought in Islam; the other three are Hanafi, Maliki, and Shafi'i schools

**haram:** anything forbidden by the Qur'an, the Sunna (actions and words of Prophet Muhammad), or the religious legal opinions of Islamic jurists, such as eating pork

**hijab**: head covering worn by some Muslim women

**hijra:** the migration of Prophet Muhammad and his followers from Mecca to Yathrib (Medina) in 622 C.E. , also known as the Hijra; Islamic calendars designate this date as year 1 A.H. (after Hijra)

**Iblis:** the Devil, Satan

**ihram:** ritual two-piece white seamless garment worn by men on pilgrimage (hajj) to Mecca, Saudi Arabia

**ijma:** consensus of the Islamic religious jurists about an issue that is not explicit in the Qur'an or the Sunna (actions and words of Prophet Muhammad)

**ijtihad** (sg.)/**istinbat** (sg.): the independent legal judgment(s) of a legal scholar

**Imam:** In Shiism, the Imam is the divinely inspired and appointed leader of the Shia community; this term is capitalized in English translations

**imam:** In Sunnism, the imam is only a religious leader; English translations do not capitalize this term

**Islam**: derives from the three Arabic root letters of s-l-m, meaning safety, security, freedom, immunity, escape, peace, submission, obedience, and gentleness

**istinja:** a ritual purity practice of using water to clean the anus and genitals after defecating or urinating

**Ithna** 'Ashariyya: the main Shia school of jurisprudence / thought

**janna:** Heaven, Paradise, or garden

**jahannam**: Hell or the Fire (nar)

**jalabiya:** an ankle- or knee-length loose-fitting garment worn by men

**janazah:** funeral prayer

**Al-Ka'ba:** a house of worship reported to have been built by prophets Abraham and Ishmael; located in Mecca, Saudi Arabia; the Prophet Muhammad ejected idols from Al-Ka'ba and rededicated it to Allah; ancient symbol of monotheism; the Sacred Mosque that all Muslims face toward in daily prayers

**kafan:** funeral shroud

**khafd:** female genital mutilation, euphemistically called circumcision

**khitan:** male circumcision

**makruh:** offensive acts, such as cigarette smoking

**Maliki:** one of the four main schools of religious jurisprudence/thought; the other three are Hanafi, Hanbali, and the Shafi'i

**mubah:** permissible religiously neutral acts, such as excessive talking

**Muslim:** a believer of Islam

**Muslimas:** female Muslims

**najis:** ritually impure

**nar:** Hellfire, also known as jahannam

**niqab:** a woman's face covering

**niyya:** the underlying aim or purpose of a person's words or actions

**qada:** decree

**qadar:** destiny

**qibla:** the direction of prayer toward the Sacred Mosque in Mecca, Saudi Arabia

**qiyas:** analogical reasoning used in creating Islamic law

**Lailatul Qadr:** The night in 610 C.E. on which Muhammad received the first revelation from God through Angel Gabriel

**Qur'an:** the revealed word of God to the Prophet Muhammad through Angel Gabriel; the holy scripture of Islam; the primary source of Islamic law

**Ramadan:** the ninth month of the year Muslims religiously observe by fasting

**rasul:** a messenger of God

**ruh:** spirit

**sadaqa**: charity

**saqt:** abortion

**salah:** ritual obligatory prayer for all Muslims performed five times daily

**sawm:** fasting during the month of Ramadan required of all able Muslims

**Shafi'i:** one of the four major Sunni schools of religious jurisprudence/thought in Islam; the other three are Hanbali, Hanafi, and Maliki

**shahadah:** the declaration of faith of Islam: "ash-hadu an la ilaha illa Llah wa ash-hadu anna Muhammadan rasulu Llah" or "I witness that there is no god but God, and I witness that Muhammad is the Messenger of God"

**shari'a:** the religious law of Islam derived primarily from the Qur'an and the words and actions of Prophet Muhammad (Sunna)

**shaykh:** a leader of a Muslim community, a respected elder, an Islamic scholar, or cleric

**Shaytan:** the Devil, Satan

**Shiism:** the second largest religious sect in Islam; founded by the followers of 'Ali ibn Abu Talib, the cousin and son-in-law of Prophet Muhammad; followers are called Shiites

**Sufism:** the mystical tradition of Islam; the practitioners of Sufism are called Sufis

**Sunna:** the words and deeds of Prophet Muhammad; his exemplary life is obligatory upon Muslims to follow

**sunna,** mandub, mustahabb, fadila, or murghab fihi: recommended acts not required of Muslims, but are best done, such as some prayers

**Sunnism:** the largest religious sect in Islam; the followers Sunnism are called Sunnis

**tawba:** repentance, turning back to God

**tahir:** ritually pure

**tawhid:** God's unity, oneness

**tayammum:** a ritual purity practice of touching a stone or clean dust with both hands, and moving the hands over the face, hands and forearms

**'ulama:** the religious community of Islamic clerics

**umma:** worldwide community of Muslims

**wudu:** ritual purity practice of washing with clean, preferably running, water the mouth, nostrils, face, hands, and forearms, wiping the head and ears, and washing the feet

**Yawm al-Qiyama:** the Final Day of Judgment

**zakah:** obligatory almsgiving to the poor

**zina:** adultery

## APPENDIX 7

# WORSHIP ITEMS

Muslims need certain items in order to fulfill their daily obligatory ritual prayer (*salah*) and other practices of their faith tradition. These items include the following paraphernalia.

1. Qur'an
2. Prayer rug (or clean towel, paper, etc.)
3. Small rock for making ritual ablution for patients unable to access running water
4. Ritual prayer (*salah*) times, which can be found at http://www.islamicity.com.
5. Large scarf for covering a woman's head along with a long-sleeved loose-fitting top and skirt
6. Kufi/topi hat for a man (optional)
7. Set of prayer beads (optional)

APPENDIX 8

# ONE HUNDRED BEAUTIFUL NAMES OF GOD

Repeating (*dhikr*) the names of God enables the reciting Muslim to turn to and surrender to God more deeply, *Insha'Allah* (God willing). The many Names of God can be a healing to the hearts, minds, souls, and bodies of believers. In Qur'an 7:180, it says, "And, God's [alone] are the attributes of perfection; invoke Him, then, by these, and stand aloof from all who distort the meaning of His attributes: they shall be requited for all that they were wont to do!" While there are 2,700 references to God in the Qur'an, the following names, qualities, or attributes of God, also from the Qur'an, are honored by Muslims worldwide.

For Muslims, reading or reciting the canonical language of Arabic is strongly encouraged. For those unable to read Arabic, however, a simple transliteration system of accents, under-dots, and underscores facilitates the reading of the Qur'an and the names of God. The transliteration guide is as follows: Read a< as in bat; i< as in beet; u <as in boot. Hold these letters two counts. Emphatic letters (h{, s{, d{, t{, dh{, and q{) are pronounced with an echo or thud.

In the name of God, The Most Gracious, The Dispenser of Grace

بسم الله الرحمن الرحيم

1. *Allāh:* The One God
2. *Ar-Raḥmān:* The All-Compassionate
3. *Ar-Raḥīm:* The All-Merciful
4. *Al-Malik:* The Absolute Sovereign
5. *Al-Quddūs:* The Holy, Pure One
6. *As-Salām:* The Source of Peace
7. *Al-Mu'min:* The Security of Faith
8. *Al-Muhaymin:* The Protector
9. *Al-'Azīz:* The Invincible
10. *Al-Jabbār:* The Omnipotent, the Compeller
11. *Al-Mutakabbir:* The Most Great
12. *Al-Khāliq:* The Creator of All
13. *Al-Bāri':* The Shaper from Nought or the Maker of order
14. *Al-Muṣawwir:* The Former of the Image
15. *Al-Ghaffār:* The Forgiver
16. *Al-Qahhār:* The Conqueror
17. *Al-Wahhāb:* The Bestower
18. *Ar-Razzāq:* The Provider
19. *Al-Fattāḥ:* The Opener
20. *Al-'Ālim:* The All-Knowing
21. *Al-Qābiḍ:* The Constrictor
22. *Al-Bāsiṭ:* The Expander

22. *Al-Bāsiṭ:* The Expander
23. *Al-Khāfiḍ:* The Abaser
24. *Ar-Rāfi':* The Exalter
25. *Al-Mu'izz:* The Venerator
26. *Al-Mudhill:* The Debaser
27. *As-Samī':* The All-Hearing
28. *Al-Baṣīr:* The All-Seeing
29. *Al-Ḥakam:* The Judge
30. *Al-'Adl:* The Just
31. *Al-Laṭīf:* The Subtle Mercy
32. *Al-Khabīr:* The Omniscient
33. *Al-Ḥalīm:* The Clement
34. *Al-'Aẓīm:* The Sublime
35. *Al-Ghaffūr:* The All-Forgiving
36. *Ash-Shakūr:* The Thankful
37. *Al-Aliyy:* The All-High
38. *Al-Kabīr:* The Vast
39. *Al-Ḥafīẓ:* The Preserver
40. *Al-Muqīt:* The Fortifier
41. *Al-Ḥasīb:* The Reckoner
42. *Al-Jalīl:* The Exalted
43. *Al-Karīm:* The Generous
44. *Ar-Raqīb:* The Watchful
45. *Al-Mujīb:* The Responder
46. *Al-Wāsi':* The Wide

47. *Al-Ḥakīm:* The All-Wise
48. *Al-Wadūd:* The Loving
49. *Al-Majīd:* The Glorious
50. *Al-Bāʻith:* The Resurrector
51. *Ash-Shahīd:* The Witness
52. *Al-Ḥaqq:* The Truth
53. *Al-Wakīl:* The Trustee
54. *Al-Qawiyy*: The Most Strong
55. *Al-Matīn:* The Firm
56. *Al-Waliyy:* The Helping Friend
57. *Al-Ḥamīd:* The Praiseworthy
58. *Al-Muḥṣī:* The Enumerator
59. *Al-Mubdi':* The Originator
60. *Al-Muʻīd:* The Restorer
61. *Al-Muḥyī:* The Giver of Life
62. *Al-Mumīt:* The Giver of Death
63. *Al-Ḥayy:* The Living
64. *Al-Qayyūm:* The Self-Subsisting
65. *Al-Wājid:* The Finder
66. *Al-Mājid:* The Glorious
67. *Al-Wāḥid:* The Unique
68. *Aṣ-Ṣamad:* The Eternal
69. *Al-Qādir:* The Decreer
70. *Al-Muqtadir:* The All-Powerful
71. *Al-Muqaddim:* The Initiator

82. *Al-'Afūww:* The Absolver
83. *Ar-Ra'ūf:* The Kind
84. *Māliku-l-Mulk:* Possessor of Sovereignty
85. *Dhū'l-Jalāli Wa'l-Ikrām:* Lord of Majesty and Bounty
86. *Al-Muqsiṭ:* The Equitable
87. *Al-Jāmi':* The Gatherer
88. *Al-Ghaniyy:* The Truly Rich
89. *Al-Mughniy:* The Enricher
90. *Al-Māni':* The Preventer
91. *Aḍ-Ḍārr:* The Harmer
92. *An-Nāfi':* The Beneficial
93. *An-Nūr:* The Light
94. *Al-Hādiy:* The Guide
95. *Al-Badī':* The Originator
96. *Al-Bāqiy:* The Everlasting
97. *Al-Wārith:* The Inheritor
98. *Ar-Rashīd:* The Spiritual Director
99. *Aṣ-Ṣabūr:* The Patient
100. *Jalla Jalālahu:* His the Majesty of Majesty

## APPENDIX 9

# ABOUT THE QUR'AN

Muslims believe that the very first revelation spoken by God through Angel Gabriel (*jibril*) to contemplative Muhammad ibn Abdullah in 610 C.E. came upon Muhammad suddenly and powerfully. The Prophet Muhammad said that, while on spiritual retreat at Mount Hira near his home in Mecca in the Arabian Peninsula,

> The angel came to him and asked him to read. The Prophet replied, "I do not know how to read." The Prophet added, "The angel caught me (forcefully) and pressed me so hard that I could not bear it any more. He then released me and again asked me to read, and I replied, 'I do not know how to read.' Thereupon he caught me again and pressed me a second time til I could not bear it any more. He then released me and again asked me to read, but again I replied, 'I do not know how to read (or what shall I read)?' Thereupon he caught me for the third time and pressed me and then released me and said, 'Read in the name of your Lord, who has created (all that exists), has created man from a clot. Read! And your Lord is the Most Generous.'" [1]

"Read in the name of your Lord, who has created (all that exists), has created man from a clot. Read! And your Lord is the Most Generous" (Qur'an 96: 1-3) were the first of 77,439 words from God, in Arabic, that the angel revealed to the unlettered Prophet Muhammad at different times and places during the last 23 years of his life.

Muslims of the seventh century C.E., during the time of the Prophet Muhammad, memorized the words of the Qur'an; some wrote the words on shards of bone, palm leaves, and rocks. Shortly after his death in 632 C.E., the successors of the Prophet Muhammad, Abu Bakr (r. 632–634 C.E.) and Uthman (r. 644-656 C.E.) compiled the revelation into book form (*mushaf*): 6,666 verses (*ayah*, sg./*ayat*, pl.) and 114 chapters (*sura*, sg./suwar, pl.). Each chapter has a name, such as "The Morning Hours" and "The Cow," and each, except chapter nine, begins with the phrase, "In the name of God, the Singularly Most Compassionate and Most Merciful" (*bismillah ar-rahman ar-rahim*). Furthermore, the 114 chapters are divided into 30 parts (*juz*). Later on, these chapters were classified according to the year and location of revelation; however, this organization of the chapters does not parallel the actual chronology of each revelation, as Muslims believe that the organization of the Qur'an belongs to God. The shorter 89 "Meccan" chapters were revealed in the first thirteen years in Mecca. These revelations were a wake-up call to the hedonistic, polytheistic Meccan society. They proclaimed the absolute unity of God, commanded their turning away from licentious conduct and toward righteous conduct and service to others, and announced the reward of Paradise or Hell according one's own deeds. The other longer 25 "Medinan" chapters were revealed in the last ten years of the life of Prophet Muhammad in Medina. They cover the rules, regulations, and guidelines of governing and of community relations, for example.

The compilation of the Qur'an more than 1,400 years ago is the same now as it was then, but translations are not. The Qur'an is the unalterable word of God, Muslims believe. The Qur'an is the uncreated word of God, scholars say. Translations, therefore, are interpretations. Translators bring their own humanness and cultural, religious, and political prejudices to the process of rendering mazes of linguistic meanings and connotations of the Arabic language of the Qur'an into other languages. Nevertheless, translations of the Qur'an are needed – given that Muslims want to understand the Qur'an in their native tongues.

Some more popular English translations of the Qur'an are as follows:

1. Abdullah Yusuf Ali, translator, *The Qur'an: Text, Translation and Commentary:* This translation is easy to read, captures some of the beautiful poetic rhythm and style of the Qur'an; provides brief chapter summaries, and has profuse footnotes.
2. Muhammad Asad, translator, *The Message of the Qur'an*: It offers a simple, straight-forward translation, generous index of names and key concepts, and extensive footnotes and explanations. All Qur'anic scripture in this handbook comes from Asad's translation.
3. Mohammed Marmaduke Pickthall, translator, *The Meaning of the Glorious Koran*: It provides an easy-to-read terse translation, brief chapter explanations, and a general index.
4. A.J. Arberry, translator, *The Koran Interpreted*: Arberry renders a translation aligned with the spirit of the original Arabic,[2] but in modern English with a poetic slant.

The Qur'an is the holiest of books in Islam. It "is the one central miracle of Islam, and this miracle of the Divine Word is actualized again and again … verbally in recitation … Its phrases are repeated in catillations at the mosque, in teaching and memorization at the mosque school and in prayers of believers."[3] The book provides the basis for the study of Muslim theology and law. Because the Qur'an is considered the unalterable Word of God, Muslims treat the book (*mushaf*, pronounced *mus-haf*) reverently. They must maintain ritual purity when touching the Qur'an, according to scholars' interpretation of Qur'an 56:77-80. In it, God says, "Behold, it is a truly noble discourse, [conveyed unto man] in a well-guarded divine writ which none but the pure [of heart] can touch: a revelation from the Sustainer of all the worlds!" Some Muslims wrap the Qur'an in beautiful cloths, kiss the Qur'an, never turn their backs on or leave the Qur'an on the floor, and most place the Qur'an on the highest shelf in a room. Qur'anic passages adorn walls, doorways, and gates of mosques, schools, homes, and other buildings, because Muslims believe the Words of God confer power and protection. Qur'an 58:21 says, "Had We bestowed this Qur'an from on high upon a mountain, thou wouldst indeed see it humbling itself, breaking asunder for awe of God." Muslims keep Qur'ans in their vehicles, at their workplaces, or in various rooms of their homes. Muslims believe that there is healing power in the words of God, which is why they recite the holy text at the bedside of their loved ones. "Thus, step by step, We bestow from on high through this Qur'an all that gives health …" (Qur'an 17:82). Muslims recite the Qur'an in Arabic (the original language of the Qur'an) daily in order to gain proximity to God and at major junctures along the continuum of existence: at the births of their children, at the bedsides of their sick or injured, and at the deaths of their loved ones. The Qur'an, Muslims believe, confers great healing power.

Muslims believe that the revelation of the Qur'an is the miracle of the prophethood of Muhammad.

---

NOTES

[1] Muhammad ibn Ismail al-Bukhari, *Sahih Bukhari.* Volume 1, Book 1, Number 3. University of Southern California *ahadith* database: http://www.usc.edu/schools/college/crcc/engagement/resources/texts/muslim/hadith/bukhari/055.sbt.html. Accessed 1 April 2010.

[2] John Gilchrist, "English Translation of the Qur'an," http://www.answering-islam.org/Gilchrist/Vol1/5d.html. Accessed 28 June 2009.

[3] Farid Esack, *The Qur'an* (Oxford: One World Publications, 2009), 18.

# BIBLIOGRAPHY

Abd-Allah, Umar Faruq. "Living Islam with Purpose." Nawawi Foundation Paper, 2007. http://www.nawawi.org/downloads/article6.pdf. Accessed 20 November 2009.

_____. "One God, Many Names." A Nawawi Foundation Paper. http://www.nawawi.org/downloads/article2.pdf, Accessed 6 April 2010.

Abdulati, Hammudah. *Islam in Focus*, rev. ed. Edited by Shaykh Salih al Husayin and Dr. Mustapha Abu Sway. Beltsville, MD: amana publications, 1998.

Abdullah, Aslam. "Real Debate about the Status of Women." The website of Islamicity.com, http://www.islamicity.com/articles/Articles.asp?ref=IC0503-2643. Accessed 3 April 2010.

Abdul-Rahman, Muhammad Saeed. *Tafsir Ibn Kathir Juz' 27* (Part 27): *Az-Zariyat 31 To Al-Hadid 29*, Part 27. London: MSA Publication, 2009.

al-Adnani, Mudher and Scheimberg, Irene. "How can we improve the rate of autopsies among Muslims?" *British Medical Journal* (4 February 2006): 310 -332.

Ahmed, W. D. "An Islamic View of Death and Dying." *Journal of the Islamic Medical Association of North America (JIMA)* 28 (1996): 175-77.

Ali, Abdullah Yusuf, trans. *The Qu'ran.* Elmhurst, NY: Tahrike Tarsile Qur'an, 1989.

Anwar, Muhammad. "Muslims in the West: demographic and socio-economic position." In *Caring for Muslim Patients,* 2nd ed. Eds. Aziz Sheikh and Abdul Rashid Gatrad. Oxon, United Kingdom: Radcliffe Publishing, 2009, 7-23.

Aramesh, Kiarash. "Abortion: An Islamic Ethical View." *Iranian Journal of Allergy, Asthma and Immunology* 6, Suppl. 5 (February 2007): 29-33.

______. "A Shiite Perspective Toward Abortion." *DARU Journal of Faculty of Pharmacy Tehran University of Medical Sciences,* No. 1 (Jan. 2006): 37-39.

Arberry, A. J., trans. *The Koran Interpreted.* London: The MacMillan Company, 1955.

Ardakani, Eslami. "Euthanasia from Christian and Islamic Points of View." *Proceedings, International Conference,* "Attitudes Towards Death in the Context of Social and Technological Changes: Challenges for Muslims and Christians." Center of Human Rights Peace and Democracy, Shahid Beheshti University, Tehran, Iran (8-10 April 2006): 31-33.

# Bibliography

Asad, Muhammad, trans. *The Message of the Qur'an.* Gibraltar: Dar al-Andalus Limited, 1980.

Askoy, S. "Making regulations and drawing up legislation in Islamic countries under conditions of uncertainty, with special reference to embryonic stem cell research." *Journal of Medical Ethics* 2005; 31: 399–403. doi: 10.1136/jme.2003.005827. http://ukpmc.ac.uk/articlerender.cgi?artid+1565514. Accessed 21 December 2009.

Assilmi, Aminah. Phone interviews conducted March 1-3, 2010, with Aminah Assilmi, (b. 1945 / d. 2010), a broadcast journalist and former director of the International Union of Muslim Women

Athar, Shahid. "Islamic Medical Ethics." *Islamic Horizons* (January - February 2002): 39-41.

______. "Contemporary Issues in the Practice of Internal Medicine." *Journal of the Islamic Medical Association of North America (JIMA)* 28 (1996): 1995-97.

______. "Ethical Decision Making in Patient Care." In *Health Concerns for Believers.* Islam-USA.com, http://74.125.113.132/search?q=cache:xJXAupqlmvwJ:www.islam-usa.com/index.php%3Foption%3Dcom_content%26view%Darticle%26id%3D349%26Itemid%3D316+%22Ethical+Decision+Making+in+Patient+Care%22+and+Shahid&cd=1&hl=en&ct=clnk&gl=us. Accessed 14 March 2010.

______. *Sex Education: An Islamic Perspective.* South Elgin, IL: KAZI Publications, 1995.

Ayoub, Mahmoud M. *Redemptive Suffering.* New York: Mouton Publishers, 1978.

Badawi, Jamal. "Is wife beating allowed in Islam?" http://www.themodernreligion.com/women/w_abuse_badawi.htm. Accessed 4 April 2010.

Blank, Jonah. "The Muslim Mainstream." In *U.S. News,* July 20, 1998, http://www.jannah.org/articles/usnews.html. Accessed 9 January 2010.

al-Bukhari, Muhammad ibn Ismail. *Sahih al-Boukhari. Being the Traditions of Sayings and Doings of the Prophet Muhammad As Narrated By His Companions,* Vol. IX. Rendered to English by Mahmoud Matraji, corrected and revised by F. Amira Zrein Matraji. Beirut, Lebanon: Dar El Aker, 1993.

al-Bukhari, Muhammad ibn Ismail. *Sahih Bukhari.* Volume 1, Book 1, Number 3. University of Southern California *ahadith* database: http://www.usc.edu/schools/college/crcc/engagement/resources/texts/muslim/hadith/bukhari/055.sbt.html. Accessed 1 April 2010.

______. *Sahih Bukhari.* Volume 3, Book 50, Number 874. University of Southern California *ahadith* database:

http;//www.usc.edu/schools/college/crcc/engagement/resources/texts/muslim/hadith/ Bukhari/050.sbt.html. Accessed 17 April 2010.

______. *Sahih Bukhari.* Volume 4, Book 52, Number 134. University of Southern California *ahadith* database: http://www.usc.edu/schools/college/crcc/engagement/resources/texts/muslim/hadith/bukhari/052.sbt.html. Accessed 4 April 2010

______. *Sahih Bukhari.* Volume 4, Book 55, Number 549. University of Southern California *ahadith* database: http://www.usc.edu/schools/college/crcc/engagement/resources/texts/muslim/hadith/bukhari/055.sbt.html. Accessed 26 December 2009.

______. *Sahih Bukhari.* Volume 4, Book 4, Number 881. University of Southern California *ahadith* database: http://www.usc.edu/schools/college/crcc/engagement/resources/texts/muslim/hadith/muslim/004.smt.html. Accessed 2 April 2010.

______. *Sahih Bukhari.* Volume 7, Book 72, Number 779. University of Southern California *ahadith* database: http://www.usc.edu/schools/college/crcc/engagement/resources/texts/muslim/hadith/bukhari/072.sbt.html. Accessed 7 December 2009.

______. *Sahih Bukhari.* Volume 8, Book 73, Number 73. University of Southern California *ahadith* database: http://www.usc.edu/schools/college/crcc/engagement/resources/texts/muslim/hadith/bukhari/055.sbt.html. Accessed 26 December 2009.

______. *Sahih Bukhari.* Volume 8, Book 75, Number 318. University of Southern California *ahadith* database: http://www.usc.edu/schools/college/crcc/engagement/resources/texts/muslim/hadith/bukhari/075.sbt.html>. Accessed 14 March 2010.

______. *Sahih Bukhari.* Volume 8, Book 75, Number 412. University of Southern California *ahadith* database: http://www.usc.edu/schools/college/crcc/engagement/resources/texts/muslim/hadith/bukhari/075.sbt.html>. Accessed 14 March 2010.

______. *Sahih Bukhari.* Volume 8, Book 75, Number 414. University of Southern California *ahadith* database: http://www.usc.edu/schools/college/crcc/engagement/resources/texts/muslim/hadith/bukhari/075.sbt.html>. Accessed 14 March 2010.

______. *Sahih Bukhari.* Volume 9, Book 42, Number 7108. University of Southern California *ahadith* database: http://www.usc.edu/schools/college/crcc/engagement/resources/texts/muslim/hadith/muslim/042.smt.html. Accessed 9 April 2010.

______. *Sahih Bukhari.* Volume 9, Book 83, Number 25. University of Southern California *ahadith* database: http://www.usc.edu/schools/college/crcc/engagement/resources/texts/muslim/hadith/bukhari/083.sbt.html. Accessed 9 April 2010.

Brockopp, Jonathan E. and Thomas Eich, eds. *Muslim Medical Ethics: From Theory to Practice.* Columbia, S.C.: University of South Carolina Press, 2008.

Carlisle, D. "Life-Giving Fatwa." *Nursing Times* 91 (1995):14-15.

Chittick, William. *The Vision of Islam.* New York: Paragon House, 1994.

Cooperson, Michael. *Classical Arabic Biography: the heirs of the prophets in the age of al-Ma'mun.* Cambridge: Cambridge University Press, 2000.

Dawood, N.J., trans. *The Koran.* New York: Penguin Books, 1986.

Dawud, Abu. *Sunan Abu Dawud,* Book 41, Number 5251, University of Southern California *ahadith* database:

http://www.usc.edu/schools/college/crcc/engagement/resources/texts/muslim/hadith/abudawud/041.sat.html. Accessed 8 December 2009.

______. *Sunan Abu Dawud*, Book 11, Number 2139, University of Southern California *ahadith* database: http://www.usc.edu/schools/college/crcc/engagement/resources/texts/muslim/hadith/abudawud/011.sat.html. Accessed 4 April 2010.

______. *Sunan Abu Dawud*, Book 28, Number 3865, University of Southern California *ahadith* database : http://www.usc.edu/schools/college/crcc/engagement/resources/texts/muslim/hadith/abudawuda/028.sat.html. Accessed 21 December 2009.

Denny, Frederick Mathewson. *An Introduction to Islam*. 2nd ed. New York: Macmillan, 1994.

Dhami, Sangeeta and Aziz Sheikh. "The family: predicament and promise." In *Caring for Muslim Patients*, 2nd ed. Eds. Aziz Sheikh and Abdul Rashid Gatrad. Oxon, United Kingdom: Radcliffe Publishing, 2009, 57-65.

Dibble, Suzanne L., Juliene G. Lipson, and Pamela A. Minarik, eds., *Culture and Nurse Care: A Pocket Guide*. San Francisco: UCSF Nursing Press, 1996.

Durrany, K.S. *Impact of Islamic fundamentalism*. Delhi: Christian Institute for the Study of Religion and Society, 1993.

Ebrahim, Abdul Fadl Mohsim. *Abortion, Birth Control and Surrogate Parenting*. Indianapolis, IN: American Trust Publications, 1989.

Ebrahimnejad, Hormoz. "Religion and Medicine in Iran: From Relationship to Dissociation." *British Journal for the History of Science* xl (2002):16.

*Encyclopaedia of Islam*, V. New Edition. Ed. C.E. Bosworth, et al. Leiden: E.J. Brill Publisher, 1986.

Esack, Farid. *The Qur'an*. Oxford, One World Publications, 2009.

Esposito, John L. and Dalia Mogahed. *Who Speaks for Islam?* New York: Gallup Press, 2007.

European Council for Fatwa and Research at http://www.islamonline.net/servlet/Satellite?pagename=Islam Online-English Ask_Scholar/FatwaE/FatwaE&cid= 1119503549272. Accessed 21 November 2009.

Fadel, Hossam E. "Assisted Reproductive Technology: An Islamic Perspective." *Journal of the Islamic Medical Association of North America (JIMA)*, 25 (1993): 14-19.

______. "Antenatal Diagnosis of Fetal Malformations: Achievements, Pitfalls, and Diagnostic Dilemmas." *Journal of the Islamic Medical Association of North America (JIMA)* 30 (1998): 99-101.

______. "The Islamic Viewpoint on New Assisted Reproductive Technologies." 30 *Fordham Urban Law Journal* (November 2002):147-58.

el-Gamel, Mahmoud A. *Islamic Finance: Law, Economics, and Practice.* New York: Cambridge University Press, 2006.

Gatrad, A.R. "Muslim customs surrounding death, bereavement, post-mortem examinations, and organ transplants." *British Medical Journal* 309 (20 August 1994): 521-3.

Gatrad, A.R., and A. Sheikh. "Medical ethics and Islam: principles and practice." *Archives of Disease in Childhood* 84 (2001):72-75.

Gatrad, Abdul Rashid and Aziz Sheikh. "Birth customs: meaning and significance." In *Caring for Muslim Patients*, 2nd ed. Eds. Aziz Sheikh and Abdul Rashid Gatrad. Oxon, United Kingdom: Radcliffe Publishing, 2009, 67-79.

al-Ghazzali, Abu Hamid Muhammad ibn Muhammad. *On Disciplining the Soul and On Breaking the Two Desires.* Translated by Timothy J. Winter. Cambridge, England: Islamic Texts Society, 1995.

______. *The Remembrance of Death and the Afterlife.* Translated by Timothy J. Winter. Cambridge, England: Islamic Texts Society, 1995.

Gilchrist, John. "English Translation of the Qur'an." http://www.answering-islam.org/Gilchrist/Vol1/5d.html. Accessed 28 June 2009.

Girshick, Lori B. *Woman-to-woman sexual violence: does she call it rape?* Boston: Northeastern University Press, 2002.

Godlas, Alan. "Islam and Islamic Studies," http://webcache.googleusercontent.com/search?q=cache:Z4vip4ZsGg8J:www.uga.edu/islam/+alan+godlas&cd=1&hl=en&ct=clnk&gl=us. Accessed 6 April 2010.

"Guidelines for Health Care Providers When Dealing with Muslim Patients." *Journal of the Islamic Medical Association of North America (JIMA)* 30 (1990): 44-45.

ter Haar, Gerrie and Yoshio Tsuruoka. *Religion and Society: An Agenda for the 21st Century.* Vol. 5, *International Studies in Religion and Society.* Leiden: E.J. Brill, 2007.

al-Hajjaj, Muslim ibn. *Sahih Muslim,* Book 4, Number 881. University of Southern California *ahadith* database: http://www.usc.edu/schools/college/crcc/engagement/resources/texts/muslim/hadith/muslim/004.smt.html. Accessed 2 April 2010.

______. *Sahih Muslim,* Volume 9, Book 42, Number 7108. University of Southern California *ahadith* database: http://www.usc.edu/schools/college/crcc/engagement/resources/texts/muslim/hadith/muslim/042.smt.html. Accessed 9 April 2010.

Hamza, Doha, compiler. *Spiritual Care Volunteer Program.* Stanford Hospital and Clinics, Muslim Spiritual Care Service at Stanford Hospital. 2006.

Hassan, Riffat. "Is Family Planning Permitted in Islam?" In *Muslim Women Scholar-activists in North America,* edited by Geisla Webb, 226-40. Syracuse, NY: Syracuse University Press, 2000.

Hassan, S. N. "Fighting to Save Life: Muslim Perspective on Health Care." *Islamic Horizons* (Jan.-Feb. 2002): 26-28.

Hathout, Hassan. "Female Circumcision Is NOT Required by Islam," at Islamic Research Foundation International, http://womanandislam.blogspot.com/2008/01/female-circumcision-2.html. Accessed 9 December 2009.

______. *Reading the Muslim Mind.* Plainfield, IN: American Trust Publications, 1995.

el-Hazmi, A.F. "Ethics of Genetic Counseling." *Annals of Saudi Medicine* 24, No. 2 (March - April 2004): 84-92.

Hedayat, Kamyar M. and Raya Pirzadeh. "Issues in Islamic Biomedical Ethics: A Primer for the Pediatrician." *Pediatrics* 108, No. 4 (Oct. 2001): 965-71.

Henley, A. and Schott, J. *Culture, Religion and Patient Care in a Multi-Ethnic Society.* London: Age Concern England, 1999.

Houtsma, M. Th. *E.J. Brill's First Encyclopaedia of Islam,* 1913-1936. Leiden: E. J. Brill, 1993.

IMANA Ethics Committee. "Islamic Medical Ethics," available at Islamic Society of North America, http://www.isna.net/Leadership/pages/Islamic-Medical-Ethics.aspx. Accessed 19 February 2010.

______. *Stem Cell Research: The IMANA Perspective.* Lombard, IL: Medical Association of North America, n.d.

International Federation of Gynecology and Obstetrics (IFGO). "Warning issued over 'unnecessary' vaginal surgery." http://www.figo.org/projects/general_assembly_resolution_FGM. Note: The IFGO passed a resolution calling for the ban of female circumcision. Visit http://www.figo.org/projects/general_assembly_resolution_FGM to view the resolution. Accessed 9 December 2009.

Islamic Society of North America (ISNA), http://www.isna.net/Leadership/pages/Islamic-Medical-Ethics.aspx. Accessed 8 January 2010.

Jonker, G. "The Many Facets of Islam: Death, dying and disposal between orthodox rule and historical convention." In *Death and Bereavement Across Cultures*, edited by C. Parkes and P. Langani, 147-65. London: Routledge, 1997.

Kathir, ibn. *Life of the Prophet Muhammad: Al-Sira Al-Nabawiyya.* Translated by Trevor Le Gassick. Reading, U.K.: Garnet Publishing, 2000.

Khan, Faroque A. "Religious Teachings and Reflections in Advance Directive – Religious Values and Legal Dilemmas in Bioethics: An Islamic Perspective." *Fordham Urban Law Journal* 30 (Nov. 2002): 147-57.

Khomeini, R. "Ruling on the final moments of life." In *Rohani M. Mogham xx I.* Tehran, Iran: Teymurzadeh Cultural Publication Foundation, 1998: 306. Rulings Nos. 1-3.

Knappert, J. "The Concept of Death and the Afterlife in Islam." In *Perspectives of Death and Dying,* edited by A. Berger, P. Badham, A.H. Kutscher, J. Berger, Michael Perry and J. Beloff. Philadelphia: T. Charles Press Publishing, 1990.

Lane, Edward William. *An Arabic-English Lexicon.* London: Williams and Norgate, 1863-93.

Mohamed Magid, president of the Islamic Society of North America, and the executive director of the All Dulles Area Muslim Society (ADAMS) in Washington, D.C. Phone interview conducted on February 10, 2010.

Malik, Imam. *Malik's Muwata.* Book 49, Number 49.3.4 University of Southern California *ahadith* database: http://www.usc.edu/schools/college/crcc/engagement/resources/texts/muslim/hadith/muwatta/049.mmt.html. Accessed 7 December 2009.

Maqsood, Ruqaiyyah Waris. *After Death, Life! Thoughts to alleviate the grief of all Muslims facing death and bereavement.* Lahore: Talha Publications, 2001.

______. *GCSE Islam.* New Dehli, India: Goodword Books, 2002.

______. *Islam*, 2nd ed. Oxford, England: Heinemann Educational Publishers, 1995.

Malik, Jamal and John R. Hinnells. *Sufism in the West.* New York: Routledge, 2006.

Mattson, Ingrid. "Adopting Children." *Islamic Horizon* January/February 2008. http://www.isnawebpaper.com/webpapers/isna0801/multi/index.html. Accessed 10 April 2010.

Memon, Kamran. "Wife Abuse in the Muslim Community." http://www.themodernreligion.com/women/w_abuse1.htm.comm. Accessed 4 April 2010.

Miklancie, Margaret A. "Caring for Patients of Diverse Religious Traditions: Islam a Way of Life for Muslims." *Home Healthcare Nurse* 25, No. 6 (June 2007): 413 – 17.

Mohaghegh, Damad S. M. "Suicide from the Viewpoint of Islamic Philosophy and Jurisprudence." *Proceedings, International Conference*, "Attitudes Towards Death in the Context of Social and Technological Changes: Challenges for Muslims and Christians." Center of Human Rights, Peace and Democracy, Shahid Beheshti University, Tehran, Iran (8-10 April 2006): 7-8.

"Muslim customs surrounding death." *British Medical Journal* 309 (20 August 1994): 521-23.

"Muslim West Facts Project." http://www.muslimwestfacts.com/mwf/125318/Religious-Perceptions-America.aspx. Accessed 6 April 2010.

Nasr, Seyyed Hossein. *The Heart of Islam*. New York: HarperCollins, 2002.

Nasr, Vali and Seyyed Vali Reza Nasr. *Forces of Fortune: The Rise of the New Muslim Middle Class and What It Will Mean for Our World.* New York: Free Press, 2009.

al-Nawawi, Yahya ibn Sharaf. *Al-Maqasid: Imam Nawawi's Manual of Islam.* Translated by Nuh Ha Mim Keller. Beltsville, MD: Amana Publications, 2002.

______. *Gardens of the Righteous.* Translated by Muhammad Zafrulla Khan. London: Curzon Press, 1989.

Neuberger, J. *Caring for Dying People of Different Faiths.* London: Mosby, 1994.

Nordin, Musa Mohd. "An Islamic Perspective of Assisted Reproductive Technologies." n.p., in online *Medical Ethics* website of the Federation of Islamic Medical Associations, http://74.125.93.132/search?q=cache:TiQ8H6AbjMYJ: www.fimaweb.net/main/medicalethics.html+%22Edwards, an+embryologist+and+Dr.+Steptoe%22&cd=4&hl= en&ct=clnk&gl=us. Accessed 8 January 2010.

Oluwasola, Olayiwola Abideen FWACP; Olufunmilayo I. Fawole, FMCPH; Abiodun Jesse Otegbayo, FWACP; Gabriel Olabiyi Ogun, FNCP;

Clement A. Adebamowo, DSc; Afolabi Elijah Bamigboye, Ph.D. "The Autopsy: Knowledge, Attitude, and Perceptions of Doctors and Relatives of the Deceased." *Pathology and Laboratory Medicine* 133, No. 1 (January 2009): 78–82.

Padela, Aasim I. "Islamic Medical Ethics: A Primer." *Bioethics* 21, No. 3 (2007): 169-78.

Pew Forum on Religion & Public Life, "Mapping the Global Muslim Population," http://webcache.googleusercontent.com/search?q=cache:wJnWS85ZuUJ:pewforum.org/WorkArea/linkit.aspx%3FLinkIdentifier%3Did%26ItemID%3D6305+mapping+the+global+muslim+population+pew&cd=1&hl=en&ct=clnk&gl=us&source=www.google.com. Accessed 22 May 2010.

Pickthall, Marmaduke, trans. *The Meaning of the Glorious Koran.* New York: New American Library, 1959.

Price, Massoume. "Rituals of Circumcision." December 2001, at the web site of Culture of Iran, http://74.125.93.132/search?q=cache:MQpXgeso55sJ:www.iranchamber.com/culture/articles/rituals_of_circumcision.php+%22Oceans+of+Light%22+and+circumcision&cd=1&hl=en&ct=clnk&gl=us. Accessed 9 December 2009.

al-Qahtanni, Sa'eed ibn Ali Ibn Wahf, compiler and referencer. *Fortification of the Muslim through Remembrance and Supplication from the Qur'an and Sunnah.* Beirut, Lebanon: Dar Ibn Hazm, 1998.

al-Qaradawi, Yusuf. *The Lawful and the Prohibited in Islam.* Translated by Kamal El-Helbawy, M. Moinuddin Siddiqui, Syed Shukry. Indianapolis, IN: American Trust Publications, 1982.

______. "Islam's Stance on Euthanasia," Islamonline.net *fatwa* databank of Qaradawi, http://www.islamonline.net/servlet/Satellite?pagename=IslamOnline-English-Ask Scholar/FatwaE/FatwaE&cid=1119503544774. Accessed 5 November 2009.

Rahman, Fazlur. *Health and Medicine in Islamic Tradition*. New York: Crossroad Publication, 1989.

______. *Islam*, 2nd ed. Chicago: The University of Chicago Press, 2002.

______. *Major Themes of the Qur'an.* Minneapolis, Minnesota: Bibliotheca Islamica, 1989.

Randhawa, Gurch. "An exploratory study examining the influence of religion on attitudes towards organ donation among the Asian population in Luton, UK." *Nephrology Dialysis Transplantation* 13 (1998): 1949-54.

Riaz, Mian N. and Muhammad M. Chaudry. *Halal food production.* Boca Raton, FL: CRC Press, 2004.

Rispler-Chaim, Vardit. *Islamic Medical Ethics in the Twentieth Century.* Leiden: E.J. Brill, 1993.

Ritter, Helmut and John O'Kane. *The Ocean of the Soul: Man, the World and God in the Stories of Farid al-Din.* Part 1, vol. 69. Translated by John O'Kane. Leiden: E.J. Brill, 2003.

Rizvi, Sayyid Muhammad. *Marriage and Morals in Islam.* Scarborough, Ontario, Canada: Islamic Education and Information Center, 1990.

Roozen, David A. "A Quick Question: How quickly are Muslim mosques growing in the U.S.?" at the website of Hartford Seminary, http://hirr.hartsem.edu/research/quick_question20.html>. Accessed 8 January 2010

al-Sadlaan, Saalih ibn Ghaanim. *Words of Remembrance and Words of Reminder: Encompassing Important Dhikr and Important Islamic Behavior.* Translated by Jamaal al-Din Zarabozo. Boulder, CO: Al-Basheer Company for Publications and Translations, 1998.

Sachedina, A. "End-of-life: The Islamic view." *Lancet* 366 (2005): 774-79.

Sachedina, Abdul. *Islamic Biomedical Ethics: Principles and Applications.* Oxford: Oxford University Press, 2009.

Sachedina, Zulie. "Islam, Procreation and the Law." *International Family Planning* 16, No. 3 (Sept. 1990): 107-11.

Saeed, Abudllah. *The Qur'an: An Introduction*. Oxford: Routledge, 2008.

Saeed, Aysha, M.D., Hartford, Connecticut. Phone interview conducted on February 2010.

Schimmel, Annemarie. *Islam: An Introduction.* Albany, New York: State University of New York, 1992.

as-Seestani, Ayatullah Ali al-Husaini. *A Code of Practice for Muslims in the West.* Translated by Sayyid Muhammad Rizvi. London, England: Imam Ali Foundation, 1999.

al-Shabrawi, Shaykh Abd Al-Khaliq. *The Degrees of the Soul.* Translated by Mostafa Al-Badawi. London: The Quilliam Press, 1987.

Sheikh, Aziz. "Death and dying – a Muslim perspective." *Journal of the Royal Society of Medicine* 91 (1998): 138-40.

Sheikh, Aziz and Gatrad, Abdul Rashid. "Death and bereavement: an exploration and a meditation." In *Caring for Muslim Patients*, 2nd ed. Eds. Aziz Sheikh and Abdul Rashid Gatrad. Oxon, United Kingdom: Radcliffe Publishing, 2009, 103-13.

Sheikh, Aziz, Gatrad, A.R., and Dhami, Sangeeta Dhami. "Culturally sensitive care for the dying is a basic human right." *British Medical Journal* 319 (1999):1073.

Siddiqi, Muzzamil and Siddiqi, Imran. "An Islamic Perspective on Stem Cell Research." http://www.islamicity.com/articles/Articles.asp?ref= IC0202-404>.Accessed 13 March 2010.

al-Sijistani, Abu Da'ud Sulayman ibn al-Ash'ath. Narrated by Abu Dawood (2792), in Abu Da'ud Sulayman ibn al-Ash'ath al-Sijistani, *Sunan Abu Dawud,* Vol. 4. Beirut, Lebanon: Dar al-Kotob al-Ilmiyah Publishing House, 2008.

Singer, P.A., D.K. Martin, and M. Kelner. "Quality end-of-life care: patients' perspectives." *Journal of the American Medical Association* 281 (1999): 163-68.

Smith, Jane I. and Yvonne Yazbeck Haddad. *The Islamic Understanding of Death and Resurrection.* New York: Oxford University Press, 2002.

Smith, Houston. *Islam: A Concise Introduction.* New York: HarperCollins, 2001.

Stork, Mokhtar. *A-Z Guide to the Qur'an: A Must-Have Reference to Understanding the Contents of the Islamic Holy Book.* Singapore: Times Books International, 1999.

Takrouri, Mohamad Said Maani and Tharwat Mohammed Halwani. "An Islamic Medical and Legal Perspective Of Do Not Resuscitate Order In Critical Care Medicine." *The Internet Journal of Health*, 7, No. 1 (2008), http://www.ispub.com/journal/the_internet_journal_of_health/volume_7_number_1_5/article/an_islamic_medical_and_legal_prospective_of_do_not_resuscitate_order_in_critical_care_medicine.html. Accessed 13 March 2010.

Veatch, Robert M. *Transplantation Ethics.* Washington, D.C.: Georgetown University Press, 2000.

Winter, Tim J. "The Muslim grand narrative." In *Caring for Muslim Patients,* 2nd ed. Eds. Aziz Sheikh and Abdul Rashid Gatrad. Oxon, United Kingdom: Radcliffe Publishing, 2009, 25-34.

Wright, John, ed. *The New York Times Almanac 2002.* New York: Penguin, 2001.

Yasin, M.N. "The End of Human Life in the Light of the Opinion of Muslim Scholars and Science." *Journal of the Islamic Medical Association of North America (JIMA)* 23 (1991): 74-81.

______. "The Inception of Human Life in the Light of the Statement from the Holy Qur'an and Sunna and the Opinion of Muslim Scholars." *Journal of the Islamic Medical Association of North America (JIMA)* 22 (1990): 159-67.

Yosef, Abdel Raheem Odeh. "Health Beliefs, Practice, and Priorities for Health Care of Arab Muslims in the United States." *Journal of Transcultural Nursing* 19, No. 3 (July 2008): 284-91.

Younis, Mohamed. "Muslim Americans Exemplify Diversity, Potential." http://www.muslimwestfacts.com/mwf/116266/ Muslim-Americans-Exemplify Diversity-Potential.aspx. Accessed 6 May 2010.